# Alternative Ageing

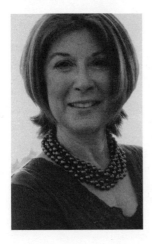

Suzi Grant worked as a broadcast journalist for over twenty years before training as a nutritional therapist. She is now a well-known health expert and nutritionist, and a member of the Guild of Health Writers and of the British Association of Nutritional Therapists. She writes regularly for health magazines and appears in the national press and on TV and radio, as well as running workshops around the country and internationally. She practises in West London and Brighton.

Her first book, *48 Hours to a Healthier Life*, was published by Penguin in 2003. She is also the author of *The Weekend Weight-Loss Plan* (previously published as *48 Hours to Kickstart Healthy Weight Loss*). You can find more information about Suzi Grant on her website: www.suzigrant.com

# Alternative Ageing

The natural way to hold back the years

## Suzi Grant

MICHAEL JOSEPH
*an imprint of*
PENGUIN BOOKS

MICHAEL JOSEPH

Published by the Penguin Group
Penguin Books Ltd, 80 Strand, London WC2R ORL, England
Penguin Group (USA) Inc., 375 Hudson Street, New York, New York 10014, USA
Penguin Group (Canada), 90 Eglinton Avenue East, Suite 700, Toronto, Ontario, Canada M4P 2Y3
(a division of Pearson Penguin Canada Inc.)
Penguin Ireland, 25 St Stephen's Green, Dublin 2, Ireland (a division of Penguin Books Ltd)
Penguin Group (Australia), 250 Camberwell Road, Camberwell, Victoria 3124, Australia
(a division of Pearson Australia Group Pty Ltd)
Penguin Books India Pvt Ltd, 11 Community Centre, Panchsheel Park, New Delhi – 110 017, India
Penguin Group (NZ), cnr Airborne and Rosedale Roads, Albany, Auckland 1310, New Zealand
(a division of Pearson New Zealand Ltd)
Penguin Books (South Africa) (Pty) Ltd, 24 Sturdee Avenue, Rosebank, Johannesburg 2196, South Africa

Penguin Books Ltd, Registered Offices: 80 Strand, London WC2R ORL, England

www.penguin.com

First published 2006
1

Set in Monotype Minion and Trinite No 2
Typeset by Rowland Phototypesetting Ltd, Bury St Edmunds, Suffolk
Printed in England by Clays Ltd, St Ives plc

A CIP catalogue record for this book is available from the British Library

ISBN-13: 978-0-718-14846-1
ISBN-10: 0-718-14846-0

# Contents

# Warning

If you are on any form of medication, chronically ill, likely to suffer an allergic reaction, or infirm in any way, please seek professional advice before trying out any treatment, exercise, herb, essential oil, food, supplement or beverage mentioned in this book. The suggestions, techniques and exercises are my personal opinions, based on my experience as a practitioner. None of them should replace medical advice or treatment.

I would also like to add that I do not receive any commission or other benefits from any of the companies whose products I have recommended throughout this book. They are simply my own suggestions for their anti-ageing benefits.

# Acknowledgements

A big thank you to all the anti-ageing experts whose books, seminars and courses have provided me with a huge amount of fascinating information and given me such a thirst for more! In particular Robert Sexauer of Isolagen, Andrew at Tree Harvest, Eric Braverman, Dr Nicholas Perricone, Brian Clement, Patrick Holford, Julia Hancock and Mary Lambert for their help and valuable contributions. To Kate Adams, Sarah Rollason, Liz Davis, Elisabeth Merriman, Keith Taylor, Catherine Hammond, Katy Nicholson and everyone at Penguin for their help and editorial improvements. To my agent Ruth for nagging me when I would much rather have been on the beach; and to all my friends and family in Brighton and beyond who've made sure I've had such fun on my days off – you know who you are and I look forward to celebrating my hundredth birthday with you all!

# Foreword

I decided to write a book on alternative ageing because I want to grow old gracefully, disgracefully and, most importantly, healthily. I spent my thirties working in TV as a chain-smoking, hard-drinking journalist. My forties brought a complete change of direction when I trained and began practising as a naturopathic nutritionist and writing health books. Now I am in my mid-fifties, I thought it about time I put everything I've learned and experienced about the ageing process together, to ensure that I, and anyone who wants to join me, enter the autumn of our lives fit, fun and for ever young. I can't expect to look like I did in my thirties, but I do expect to *feel* like I did: full of life, enthusiasm, energy, vitality and glowing with health. There is enough evidence from anti-ageing doctors and gerontologists to suggest that there is no reason why we can't remain physically and mentally active till at least a hundred and beyond. I want to be one of those people.

I am lucky enough to live in the seaside city of Brighton & Hove where it is totally acceptable to be a fit seventy-something who swims in the sea all year round. If you want to go clubbing at fifty, that's fine; it's OK to take up roller-blading at sixty. No one treats you as if you should be tucked up at home with your cat and slippers. It's all a state of mind, and, as you will find out, we can all look younger and healthier and *feel* younger and healthier if we follow our hearts and stop worrying about what we should and shouldn't be doing at a certain age.

Yes, I get more tired than I used to. Yes, I have more wrinkles and slacker skin. But, so far, I have avoided all the aches, pains and degenerative illnesses that people think it is normal to suffer at my age. And I intend to carry on avoiding them. The secret of healthy ageing isn't medical intervention or surgery but the food we eat, our lifestyle and the attitude we have to life. So I have put together an alternative ageing plan that, I hope, will encourage you to join me dancing on the beach when I'm ninety.

I dedicate this book to all baby boomers everywhere. May we all age healthily, youthfully and disgracefully!

# Introduction

A baby boomer, apparently, is anyone born between 1946 and 1964 – anyone from fortyish to sixty. We're a lucky generation. We seem to have led the way since the Swinging Sixties. We *invented* sex, drugs and rock 'n' roll, for goodness' sake. Then we got sensible and launched ourselves into a frenzy of bringing up kids and rising to the top of our careers. We power-dressed our way through the eighties, and then found ourselves, in the words of Shirley Conran, too busy to stuff a mushroom!

Now we are discovering a different way of being middle-aged. We are finding out that entering our third age can be a wonderful time to discover a *new* age and a more spiritually aware, less material, downsized life. The children have grown up and flown the nest, some of us are single again, or widowed, some of us have retired while others will work till they drop. But none of us is prepared to enter middle or old age like our mothers did: there will be no blue rinses or sensible shoes for us. We want to stay healthy and feel and look younger than our biological age – naturally. And if we can find a perfect work/life balance with a bit of spirituality and good health thrown in, and have a lot of fun, then we really can look forward to a long and happy life.

No one looks forward to growing old: our immune system doesn't work as well as it once did, our bones get weaker and our organs wear out. At the same time our percentage of body fat increases and everything starts heading south. However, with a change in attitude, lifestyle and especially nutrition, you can look forty at fifty, fifty at sixty and sixty at eighty without resorting to cosmetic surgery. You will still age but you'll age *more slowly*. Ageing is inevitable, but ageing badly and unhealthily isn't.

I hope this book will empower you to do whatever it is you

want to do with the rest of your life. Taking you through twelve easy steps to alternative ageing, you will find an answer to all the questions women our age ask.

*Top Ten Questions*
1. How do I sail through the menopause? (See pages 44–9)
2. What are the best anti-ageing foods? (See page 50)
3. What are the best anti-ageing supplements? (See page 126)
4. How can I beat middle-age spread? (See pages 152–3)
5. How can I have younger-looking skin? (See page 163)
6. How can I sleep better? (See page 203)
7. How can I improve my sex drive? (See pages 213–14)
8. How can I protect my bones and joints? (See page 148)
9. How can I have more energy? (See page 196)
10. What am I going to do with the rest of my life? (See pages 220–1)

*Alternative Ageing* will guide you through a crash course in living long and healthily. I have tried everything I recommend in the book and hope you have as much success as I have had following the twelve key steps, so you too can look and feel the very best you can – from the inside out and the outside in.

Super Agers – what ages you, inside and out
Super Hormones – healthy glands equal happy hormones
Super Foods – the best anti-ageing foods
Super Fats – why essential fats are anti-ageing
Super Drinks – the best anti-ageing drinks, including anti-ageing juices and smoothies
Super Anti-Ageing Diet – a choice of diets and how to Eat for Life
Super Supplements – the best anti-ageing supplements
Super Bod – from healthy hair to fabulous feet
Super Skin – what's on offer and alternatives to do at home
Super Fit – which exercises keep you young
Super Life – you are never too old to change your life
Super Anti-Ageing Day – how to make your day as anti-ageing as possible

But first, a check list. Statistically, people who rate well on each of the following points have the best chance of living longer than average. You should use the results in conjunction with a complete physical examination by your GP before embarking on your new alternative ageing regime. Then follow the advice in this book.

10  is excellent
5  is average
0  is below average

## How Well Am I Ageing?

*Cardiovascular Disease*

How many of your parents and/or grandparents suffered a heart attack or stroke before 60?

None  10
One or two  5
Three or more  0

*My Last Cholesterol Reading Was*

Excellent (under 200mg)  10
Average (220mg)  5
Poor (over 240mg)  0

*My Last BP Reading Was*

Excellent (120/70)  10
Fair (130/90)  5
Poor (140/95 or higher)  0

*Job Satisfaction*

When I go to work in the morning, I feel:

Eager for new challenges  10
Ready to do the job, but not excited  5
Uninterested – it's only a job  0

*Cigarette Smoking*

Over the last 5 years I have:

Never smoked  10
Smoked occasionally  5
Smoked regularly  0

*Physical Fitness*

Breathing, circulation, etc., compared to 10 years ago

I feel almost exactly the same  10
I notice a few things wrong  5
I have a medical condition  0

*Happiness*

All things considered, my life these days is:

Very fortunate  10
Pretty good most of the time  5
About as good as the next person's  0

*Self-health Rating*

This year my general health has been:

Excellent  10
Good  5
Fair or poor  0

*General Intelligence*

On IQ tests I come out:

Above average (120 and over)  10
Average (100–110)  5
Below average (90 or below)  0

A score of 90 indicates you are likely to live longer than the national average. An above-average score (65–90) suggests you should live at least three years longer than the norm, more if you are already past middle age. A below-average score (45–65) indicates you need to pay more attention to your health and well-being.

If you are over fifty a score of 75–90 indicates a likelihood of long life. The same score would not be as significant if you were only thirty!

I got 80! Great news. How did you do?

# 1.

# Super Agers

Let's start with what actually ages you: the external and internal factors that can make you unhealthy and old before your time. Super Agers are what I consider to be the enemies of a youthful old age and to be avoided as much as possible if you want to age healthily and beautifully!

## Free Radicals

One of the major contributors to ageing is free radicals, due to the damage they do to the body's cells. The reaction between free radicals and DNA is thought to contribute to many forms of cancer, and they may also be involved in promoting Parkinson's and Alzheimer's disease, arthritis, diabetes, heart disease and many other illnesses. Free radicals are unstable molecules lacking electrons. They steal electrons from stable molecules, turning those molecules into free radicals and setting off a chain reaction. Normally the body copes with its free radicals through antioxidants which donate electrons to them. But free radicals increase with age and there could be millions of them by the time we're fifty. Watch a piece of fruit when it's cut and left out in the air – it appears to rust. That's what happens to your cells without enough antioxidants. Although a healthy diet full of antioxidants and a strong immune system will repair most of the damage, what is left accumulates. So we need to take steps to prevent free radical invasion if we want to stop the body from ageing rapidly.

Professor Denham Harman, from the University of Nebraska Medical School, gained international acclaim as the father of the free-radical theory of ageing. 'The chances are 99 per cent that free radicals are the basis for ageing. These oxidants, produced by the body every time we turn glucose into energy, eventually kill us. If we take in more oxidants by smoking or living surrounded by toxins and consume few antioxidants, we will age even quicker.'

## Toxins

Toxins can be poisonous, harmful, deadly, harm*less* or just ageing because their presence encourages even more free-radical pro-duction. Although many medical experts don't believe toxins exist, most anti-ageing experts do. Like me, they consider *anything* that gets into the cells and causes an imbalance to be a toxin. Our bodies should be able to cope, but even the strongest system can be weakened by a constant toxic onslaught especially the adrenal and thyroid glands. We live in a fog of toxic chemicals, from herbicides and fungicides in our food to solvents in our homes and offices. From air pollution to pain killers, a toxin doesn't necessarily have to be something 'poisonous', just something we breathe in, ingest or touch that our body does not recognize as a 'friend'. The more unnatural the component, the more unlikely it is to match our own molecules and the more cleansing work the cells have to do to keep you healthy and young.

The fight against much of your body's free radical production will be won by the foods suggested in the Super Foods chapter (see page 50). But for a really good kick-start have a look at these lists of what I call toxins and see how many are ruling your life and health. Some of them will surprise you. Some of them are imposs-ible to live without, unless you go and live on top of a mountain on your own! However, most of them produce the free radicals that age us, or are extremely stressful to the body which also ages us – so they're worth at least a read for the sake of your health and your skin!

# Internal Agers

## Unhealthy Foods

*Fried food*
*Processed food*
*Fast food and takeaways*
*Non-organic food*

## The Three Ss

*Salt*
*Sugar*
*Stimulants: coffee, tea, alcohol*

## Drugs

*Cigarettes*
*Prescription drugs*
*Over-the-counter medicine*
*Social drugs*

## Acidic Foods

*Wheat*
*White rice*
*Dairy*
*Meat*
*The potato and its relatives*

# External Agers

*Sunbathing*
*Air pollution*
*Regular airline travel*
*Regular tube or metro travel*
*Regular mobile phone use*
*Electrical equipment*
*Chemicals*

## Emotional Agers

*Unhealthy relationship*
*Stressful job*
*Stressful home life*
*Little or no exercise*
*Little or no fresh air or sunlight*
*Always on the go*
*Don't meditate*
*Don't do breathing exercises*
*Don't do yoga or tai chi*
*No time to just sit and be*
*No time to relax*
*No time for 'me'*

As far as this last list is concerned, it all adds up to one big fat word – stress! The rest of the book will take care of most of these stressers, especially the Super Life chapter on page 202, but first a quick romp through *why* these Super Agers need to be addressed.

## Internal Agers

*Fried Food*
Apart from the fact that most fried food is extremely high in saturated fat which can lead to furred-up arteries, high cholesterol and heart disease, frying makes the oils or fats used (apart from the ones mentioned in Super Fats on page 78) unstable and potentially hazardous. As they break down they cause free radicals to run riot around the body.

*Processed Food*
One of Britain's leading food authorities, Dr Erik Millstone, who is involved in science and technology research at Sussex University, estimates that no fewer than *four thousand* additives are used in packaged food and drinks in the UK today. He has calculated that

an average person eating an average diet consumes 6–7 KILOS of additives a year!

Processed food is more likely to be loaded with salt or sugar or both – especially low-fat foods. If the fat is taken out of foods it is usually replaced by salt or sugar to make it tasty. Nothing ages you more quickly than eliminating the right fats from your diet, but more of that later in the Super Fats chapter. There is also a lot more on the horrors of salt and sugar coming up (see pages 12 and 14).

### Fast Food and Takeaways

Although partial to the odd Indian meal myself, takeaways are definitely more prone to be loaded with salt or sugar. Fast food may not always be full of additives but it may still be extremely high in saturated fat and short on fibre and enzymes – two essentials for a youthful appearance.

Fast food can also be very hard to digest and could add to your toxic load by staying in the colon far longer than a home-cooked meal. The longer the food stays in the colon, the more it begins to rot and produce toxins which get absorbed into the bloodstream and taken to every cell in the body.

### Non-Organic Food

'Eating non-organic produce is like taking part in a long-term experiment, swallowing something like *one gallon* of pesticides and organophosphates a year,' warns Roz Kadir, a nutritionist who specializes in sports nutrition.

Chemicals added to your food are known as hormone disruptors and can affect the function of every cell in your body and accelerate ageing.

Be aware, though, that an organic label doesn't always mean 'healthy'. An organic pizza, for example, is still full of saturated fat and salt. Only some of the pizza's ingredients need to be organically grown for it to be allowed an organic label, so don't be conned into thinking that just because food is labelled organic it's healthy and will give your body the best nutrition.

## The Three Ss

### Salt

Excess sodium chloride, or salt, increases blood pressure, is linked to heart disease and stroke and even osteoporosis and stomach cancer. Too much salt encourages the body to hang on to water for dear life causing bloating and water retention. It is vital for our metabolism and electrolyte balance, and without it we would certainly die, but we only need about 6 grams a day and most of us consume twice that amount.

Eighty per cent of the salt that we eat comes from salt hidden in foods, for example processed, restaurant, fast and canteen food.

Professor Graham MacGregor of St George's Hospital in London is a leading expert on the relationship between salt and cardio-vascular disease and says that reducing salt intake from the 10–12g a day currently consumed to the recommended intake of 5–6g a day would save approximately 70,000 people from suffering strokes and heart attacks each year – half of which are fatal. 'We need to be much more aware of all the salt that is hidden in food – classic examples are things like cornflakes which are almost as salty as seawater and contain more salt than crisps. Bread is also a major source of salt in the UK diet.' These are the foods to be very wary of and if you're not sure how to measure the sodium content here is a tip for perusing those labels.

TOP TIP: READING THE LABELS

> *If the labelling states 5 grams of salt per 100 grams, you know what you're getting. But if it says sodium, you need to do a bit of maths! Whatever the sodium amount shown, multiply by 2.5 to find out the actual salt content. You might be quite shocked.*

### WORST SALT OFFENDERS LIST

- *Bacon*
- *Smoked or cured meat like ham*
- *Baked beans*

- *Margarine*
- *Hard cheese like Cheddar*
- *Breakfast cereals*
- *Biscuits*
- *Pizza*
- *Potato crisps*
- *Ready meals*
- *Sausages*
- *Smoked fish: just 50g of smoked salmon contain more than 3.75g of salt!*
- *Tinned soups*
- *Tomato ketchup*
- *White bread: one sandwich contains half the recommended daily allowance (RDA) in just the bread* without *the filling.*

The anti-ageing diets will automatically reduce your sodium intake by as much as 80–85 per cent. You will still consume the recommended daily allowance for sodium, but in an organic, absorbable form – green vegetables, for example, are full of sodium. If you find your food really bland without salt, don't worry, you can use a little unrefined sea salt or crystal salt (see page 74) with my blessing.

Meanwhile, try and cut down salt as much as possible. It's amazing how quickly your taste buds will adapt to finding foods such as takeaways too salty.

TOP TIPS

*Stop adding salt to your cooking.*
*Stop adding salt to your food without tasting it first.*
*Cut right down on tinned, pickled or smoked foods.*
*Cut right down on ready-made meals, especially low-fat ones.*
*Read the labels very carefully and look for the sodium content.*
*Remember that the RDA is just 6g of salt which equals one teaspoon.*
*Within 2–6 weeks you won't want it any more.*

*Sugar*
Ninety per cent of people who have Candida got it from excess sugar.

An excess of refined sugar shortens your lifespan and ages you because it robs your body of vital vitamins and minerals, prevents essential fats from being utilized, feeds the gut's bad bacteria, causing bloating and, eventually, Candida, and dissolves the minerals in our teeth. Sugar also puts stress on the adrenal glands and interferes with insulin function causing fluctuating blood-sugar levels. Sugar plays no part in an anti-ageing programme because, according to the experts, it crosslinks with proteins, stiffening tissue, making it less flexible and elastic and causing wrinkles. This process is called glycation.

Sugar has no nutritional value whatsoever. Yes, it is lovely and it's moreish. But that craving for a chocolate bar mid-afternoon is just a dip in blood-sugar levels. The more sugar you eat, the more highs and lows you are going to experience in your blood-sugar. If the glucose produced by eating that sugary snack has nowhere to go, the body simply lays it down as fat.

As for artificial sweeteners, they also play no part in an anti-ageing plan. We don't know enough about the long-term effects of the chemicals used to make them and, as far as I'm concerned, they have had enough bad press to be considered toxins.

Finally, soft drinks. They leach calcium out of the bones and also raise blood-sugar levels, increase insulin production and turn you into a fat-producing machine. The more you drink sweetened drinks, even if they are artificially sweetened, the more you will crave carby, sugary snacks. More importantly, whether they are low cal or 'full fat', many of them contain additives and colourings such as formaldehyde, aspartic acid and phenylalanine. More on super-ageing chemicals later (see page 26).

*Stimulants: Coffee*

Drinking just two cups of coffee a day can increase levels of the ageing hormone cortisol. Cortisol is one of the two hormones that increase with age, so we need to keep consumption of coffee well under control. Excessive coffee drinking can also affect the immune system, brain cells, insulin production and, surprisingly, cause weight gain. No one knows why, but clinical studies show that by reducing coffee intake body fat goes down, especially if it is replaced by green tea. (More of that later in the chapter on Super Drinks.)

Caffeine is also the most active stimulant for the nervous system. It can cause insomnia, digestive and bowel problems and can even affect the heart. It is a very strong diuretic, is dehydrating and, in excess, can really dry those cells out. Not good news if you want plumped-up skin.

If coffee is not organically grown, many toxic chemicals are used when it is being produced. 'Decaf' coffee is even worse, because chemicals such as methylene chloride or trichlorethylene are used to decaffeinate the coffee. If you drink decaf make sure it has been prepared by the 'water or Swiss process', which means steam distillation has been used to remove the caffeine.

However, as a bit of a coffee addict myself, I appreciate how difficult it is to cut out. In moderation, it is a wonderful pick-me-up and my favourite stimulant, especially while writing! But I do stay off it for many months at a time and find it very easy if I drink green tea instead. If you really can't live without coffee, make it just one, organic cup a day.

Caffeine also leaches calcium and B vitamins out of the body, so you need to make sure you eat plenty of the Super Foods high in these nutrients (see page 50), if you want to continue drinking coffee.

*Stimulants: Tea*

Tea, on the other hand, has been getting some good press recently. Britain's favourite beverage is full of antioxidants that fight ageing and free radicals. Tea also contains an amino acid called theanine, which increases levels of dopamine, the feel-good brain chemical.

But (there's always a but isn't there?) tea is still a diuretic, dehydrating and challenging to the body if it is full of milk and sugar. An excess of tea can also inhibit iron absorption. So think about reducing your intake to a couple of cups a day of the best, really high-quality tea. Or, better still, try one of the many alternative teas recommended under Super Drinks (see page 101).

*Stimulants: Alcohol*

Alcohol, strictly speaking, is not a stimulant because it depresses the nervous system. But it does stimulate the liver, causes insomnia and is very dehydrating so is bound to be ageing. Just think of that thumping headache the morning after the night before. It's due to dehydration caused by water rushing away from your brain to go and deal with your overworked kidneys. If you want a nice plumped-up skin, cut it right down.

Remember that alcohol contains sugar and is stored by the body as fat. Drinking too much will play havoc with your blood-sugar levels as well as adding another spare tyre round your middle.

If you wondered, as I have for a long time, why you wake up in the middle of the night after drinking, there is a very good reason. Scientists know that after the alcohol sends you off to sleep, it precipitates a burst of norepinephrine, a hormone that increases as a result of excitement or stress. So, hours after drinking, your body releases a burst of norepinephrine and you're wide-awake at three in the morning. If you want to sleep well, and benefit from all the skin repairing that goes on during the night, keep alcohol to a minimum.

Red wine is my poison and I do justify it by acknowledging that it is rich in antioxidants that have recently been linked to the low rates of heart disease in France. But I am talking about one or two glasses occasionally, not every night.

TOP TIP

*The average body needs approximately 4–5 molecules of water for every molecule of alcohol drunk to help remove it from the body. So drink 1–2 glasses of water for every glass of booze you drink to help your hydration levels.*

## Drugs

### Cigarettes

The hardest of all drugs to give up: scientists constantly warn us that if you don't stop smoking you can expect to die ten years earlier than your non-smoking friends. We all know the killer diseases cigarette smoking cause, but it also ages your skin quicker than any other toxin. One puff of cigarette smoke produces thousands of free radicals in our lungs, which then circulate throughout the body affecting every cell, gland and organ, making your skin lined and your teeth yellow! Enough said.

Even if you don't smoke or smoke very few cigarettes, don't sit in smoky places. Secondary smoke is also very toxic. As your friend sits considerately holding her fag in the air in between puffs, the smoke is going straight into your lungs, laden with those toxic chemicals. The smoke she blows *out* isn't half as toxic because she's inhaled most of them.

If you can't get your partner to give up, at least make him or her smoke outside. It has been found that pets in smoking households die younger, so imagine what it's doing to you.

If you are still smoking by the time you get to the end of this book, make it one of your lifestyle changes and plan to see a hypnotherapist, a doctor for nicotine-replacement therapy, or anyone who can help you give up – for good!

*Prescription Drugs*

I am not suggesting for one minute that you throw away any pre-scription drugs you need for a life-threatening or chronic condition. But do bear in mind that all drugs, legal or illegal, herbal or pharma-ceutical, have some toxicity and the liver has to deal with them. An overworked liver can't help you beat ageing.

*Over-the-Counter Medicines*

If you constantly take over-the-counter treatments for headaches, backache, constipation or indigestion try to do without them for a few weeks to give your liver a chance to repair itself. It only takes six weeks for the liver to completely regenerate itself, and you will soon notice an improvement to your skin. You will read more about how to look after the liver in Super Bod (see page 155) and there are plenty of alternative remedies for any niggling, not-so-serious ageing problems you may have throughout the rest of the book.

In the meantime, just consider this. Dr Simon Ellis, a con-sultant neurologist at North Staffordshire Hospital, says that if you take bought painkillers on more than seven days every month it's *excessive* for your liver's health.

*Social Drugs*

As a baby boomer you may well still roll a joint occasionally. It may be a 'herb', but marijuana includes tetrahydrocannabinol, which just gets stored in the body fat and liver causing more free-radical production. Any social drug taken habitually needs at least one annual detox.

## Acidic Foods

Although acidic foods aren't really 'toxins' they do create a chal-lenge for the body if eaten in excess. The greater the challenge, the more dehydrated and stressed the cells become. If the body is challenged constantly over a long period it becomes very 'dry'; the stomach won't easily digest everyday foods, and the liver won't be able to do its job properly. The result: poor skin, bloating, lethargy, constipation, joint problems, arthritis and more. All things we want to avoid if we are to look and feel full of life and vigour.

Challenging foods take an enormous amount of the digestive system's energy to get broken down, used or thrown out. The more complicated the meal, the more energy is needed, and the more lethargic we feel as blood is shunted away from places like the brain to go to work on the digestive process. The gastro-intestinal tract (your gut) becomes clogged and full of stagnating food and the thousands of little finger-like projections in your small intestines (villi) can't absorb the food properly and dis-ease sets in.

Dis-ease, in this context, is acidity in the cells. If the cells are too acidic they cannot get rid of toxins or acids easily and won't absorb essential minerals and nutrients, and you'll age badly. I won't go into detail about pH levels of acidity and alkalinity except to say that the body produces both acid and alkaline fluids. The stomach should be acidic while bile and pancreatic juice should be alkaline. Together they neutralize the stomach's contents as it comes through the small intestine.

Because of our diet, most of us are acidic where we should be alkaline and alkaline where we should be acidic. So here is a brief reminder of what foods are particularly acidic and why you should cut down your consumption if you want to age well. You will find most of them missing from the Super Foods chapter for the reasons I have mentioned, but it doesn't mean you must never have a bread roll or a lump of cheese if you want to, it just means be aware of each food's disadvantages and make up your own mind.

*Wheat*
Although whole-grain wheat is a good source of complex carbo-hydrate and gives your body healthy amounts of vitamins and minerals, it is very challenging, hard to digest and acidic. Most of the bread on supermarket shelves tends to be poor quality: full of sugar, salt and additives. If you need proof of how many additives a cheap loaf contains, just see how long it lasts in your fridge compared to a French, freshly baked baguette that goes stale in a

matter of hours. English bread is blamed for more digestive and bowel problems than any other food. It is very interesting to note how many of my clients have absolutely no problem with wheat when they are on holiday out of the UK!

Latest figures from the organization Allergy UK show that while 20 per cent of the UK's population think they are suffering from a wheat intolerance, less than 3 per cent really are. Going by my own clients, I think that figure could be much higher.

Many people suffer from wheat intolerance because of the gluten in bread. Two insoluble proteins in glutinous grains, called gliadins and glutenins, produce gluten when the flour is kneaded with water. It makes bread-making possible but it is also the gliadin part of the mixture that appears to cause gluten intolerance, irritating the colon in a great many people. Gliadin can coat the wall of the colon, upset the bowel flora and prevent absorption, all of which can lead to constipation, discomfort, putrid bacteria, bloating, lethargy and IBS, as well as other more serious bowel disorders such as Celiac or Crohn's disease.

Even if you suffer from none of the above, every time you eat a sandwich or a bowl of pasta your body needs the equivalent of three cups of water to be able to convert the starch to glycogen to be stored. As a result, your waistline expands and you hit a huge energy slump.

If you think you may be intolerant to wheat, you will find many alternatives in the Super Foods chapter. But if you have a robust digestion that can cope with bread then fine, go ahead and eat it. If you're not sure, read the rest of the book first, especially Super Bowels (page 153), in the Super Bod chapter. If you suffer from bloating and are not going to the loo as often as you should, you shouldn't be eating wheat!

My personal take is that a truly hydrated body will not have a problem with whole-grain wheat occasionally – not four times a day. If you know you are going to have a very wheaty meal, make sure you drink a pint of water an hour or more beforehand to help it on its way.

*White Rice*
White rice has the healthiest part of the grain containing all the B vitamins stripped away in the processing. It is usually bleached, cleaned, pearled (polished with talc), oiled and coated. It may be more digestible than wheat but there is little nutrition in it. Replace it with the much healthier, nutrient-rich grains recommended in Super Foods.

*Dairy*
Dairy, in my world, is milk and cheese from cows as opposed to goats or sheep. Butter and yogurt from cow's milk are fine. Food intolerance and allergy to dairy is very common in the UK, and as many as 8 per cent of all white Europeans suffer from it. A whopping 80 per cent of Africans, as well as many Asians, and their descendants, cannot tolerate dairy at all due to a lack of the milk-sugar digesting enzyme, lactase.

If you suffered from chronic ear infections, tonsillitis, eczema or asthma as a child you may well be sensitive to the proteins and sugars in cow's milk. Lactose and milk casein are the two most common offenders. Milk is also very mucus forming, as well as being acidic, and has long been associated with chronic catarrh, sinusitis and hay fever.

Skimmed milk isn't much better than whole milk. Although the saturated fat has been removed, the vitamins A and D have also been removed. All that calcium you think you are getting from milk needs vitamin D, as well as magnesium, to help absorption.

Boiled milk is, however, more digestible than cold milk and is also full of tryptophan which aids relaxation and sleep. So if you can't go without your nightly cup of hot milk or cocoa, at least make sure it is organic and semi-skimmed or full fat.

We are the only mammals on the entire planet that drink milk as adults. Every other fully grown mammal gets calcium from the dark green vegetation they eat. The highest rates of osteoporosis are found in the countries that consume the most milk. There are plenty of alternatives for you in the chapter on Super Foods, such as goat's cheese, green vegetables and almonds – they provide as much calcium as milk, if not more, and in a more absorbable form. You won't be going without dairy completely either as I have snuck in a few surprises.

If you are fine with dairy and don't suffer from any of the aforementioned conditions, then do carry on. But please, first, consider some dairy facts:

## DAIRY FACTS

- *Cheese has very high sodium levels*
- *Cheese is extremely hard to digest*
- *Casein is the same substance used to make one of the strongest wood glues known*
- *Cheese causes excessive mucus in the intestines*
- *Cheese encourages putrid bacteria to live in the intestine*
- *Cheese affects mineral absorption*
- *Cows may be fed antibiotics and hormones, which are then passed on to you*
- *Most of the nutrients in milk fat are lost in the pasteurizing process*
- *Milk contains approximately ten times more calcium than magnesium, a complete imbalance, which can lead to health problems*

*Meat*

A diet high in saturated fat from foods such as bacon, sausages and processed meat will almost certainly lead to higher cholesterol levels and heart disease. Meat is very acidic and can also encourage the growth of unfriendly bacteria, causing bloating and constipation. It can take *days* to get a thick, juicy steak digested and out of the body.

Unless they have been organically raised, the animals may have been fed hormones and antibiotics and eaten grass contaminated by pesticides. Studies suggest that vegetarians enjoy ten more years of disease-free living than meat eaters and are less likely to die from cancer and heart disease. On the other hand, animal protein is absolutely essential for cell and tissue health and youthful skin.

A lack of offal in our diet is said to be a contributing factor to the epidemic of under-functioning thyroids we are now seeing. But anyone with a history of arthritis, bowel cancer or heart disease should try and replace some of their meat meals with healthier, oily fish, if you can. There is a lot more information on the benefits of protein in the Super Foods chapter, so wait till you have read that before you decide whether you need to cut down your meat consumption or not.

Meanwhile, here is a list of meats, going from best to worst, for your long-term health. As you will see when you get to the Super Meats section on page 62, if you want to continue eating meat, buy the best quality, organic meat you can find and you will need to worry less about this list, apart from maybe the last point.

## MEAT AGERS

- *Game*
- *Poultry*
- *Lamb*
- *Beef*
- *Pork*
- *Offal*
- *Meat products: sausages, bacon, ham*

### The Potato and its Relatives

Potatoes are on the Super Agers list because, much like wheat, they require an enormous amount of water to be digested, because they contain so much starch. Although they are a highly nutritious, fibre-packed carbohydrate, they can be very hard work for some people.

Anyone who suffers from blood-sugar problems should treat potatoes as an occasional treat. A baked potato, for example, can release its sugar and starch content very fast, pushing glucose levels in the blood too high and too quickly, triggering inflammation and fatigue. Boiled potatoes are better than baked or mashed for anyone suffering from blood-sugar fluctuations.

Which brings us on to the final reason for some of you to avoid potatoes and their relatives. Potatoes, tomatoes, aubergines, courgettes and peppers all belong to the Solanaceae family and contain a substance called solanine. It is well known that anyone suffering from arthritis and other inflammatory conditions can have a dramatic reduction in pain when they avoid any of the foods from the nightshade family. Whether this is due to the solanine or the acidity of these foods remains to be seen. But for anyone in pain, it is certainly worth excluding the nightshade family from your diet and seeing if it makes any difference.

For anyone else, all of the above vegetables have certain health benefits and, apart from potatoes, are certainly good for their anti-ageing properties.

## External Agers

### Sunbathing

When it comes to anti-ageing, there is a huge amount of information about why we shouldn't sunbathe and why we *should* in the Super Skin chapter (see page 164). Meanwhile, to state the obvious: too much sun wrinkles your skin, causes permanent damage to skin cells and can lead to skin cancer. If you want younger-looking skin stay out of the sun between 11 a.m. and 3 p.m. in the summer.

### Air Pollution

Air pollution in our cities and towns is now commonly associated with the rise in asthma and other bronchial conditions. Imagine what it's doing to your skin, internally and externally. You can protect yourself from the free radicals and toxicity produced by increasing your intake of fruit and veg from the Super Foods lists (pages 54 and 58).

*Regular Airline Travel*

I know there's not a lot you can do about this one but here is what your poor body is exposed to on a long flight: ozone and radiation at high altitudes, lack of oxygen, jetlag, stress and a risk of deep vein thrombosis (DVT). When you fly avoid all 3 Ss – salt, sugar, stimulants – and drink more water. Your cells need a minimum of the recommended 2 litres a day when you are travelling long haul. Book an aisle seat so you can get to the loo easily and stretch your legs in between the trolley runs.

*Regular Tube or Metro Travel*

London's Underground system is high in lead, asbestos and all manner of chemicals as well as electromagnetic waves. Nowadays travelling by tube is also extremely stressful. Take a bus, cycle or walk. There are more tips on how and why to walk wherever and whenever you can in the Super Fit chapter.

*Regular Mobile Phone Use*

This one makes me very angry, even as I type! What happened to the true meaning of 'mobile'? They are supposed to be used when we are *mobile*, not for long chats at home. And if you use the word 'cell' phone instead, just consider this: spending just thirty seconds on a mobile or cell phone is enough to open up your blood-brain barrier, which protects your brain 'cells' from toxins, *for 8 hours*. Cut down on your use of the mobile and turn it off when you're at home. It will keep your brain younger!

*Electrical Equipment*

*All* electrical appliances, including this laptop that I am living in front of at the moment, emit electromagnetic fields (EMFs). Some of them give off even higher levels than those found under the most powerful overhead transmission line. According to Jean Philips, of Powerwatch, 'Many scientists believe the EMFs around may be damaging our health, weakening our immune system and encouraging diseases like cancer and Alzheimer's.'

Even a few minutes a day can lead to depression, headaches,

mood swings, low energy and poor concentration, according to Powerwatch. Tell me about it. I felt muggy-headed, drained and *looked* completely dehydrated after a few hours working on my computer, until I got some advice. Help is at hand in the Super Life chapter (see page 202) where you will find a selection of plants and other things that help protect you against the 'electro smog' surrounding us.

*Chemicals*
Apart from the chemicals that may be hidden in our food and drink there are also thousands that we may be putting on our skin, the body's largest organ. Much of what you put on your skin is absorbed and taken into the bloodstream so, wherever possible, try and change to natural, chemical-free products for the sake of your and your family's health. Here's a list of the more frightening Super Agers that are commonly found in your everyday cosmetics and household items:

## SKIN TOXINS

- *Collagen: found in skin products. Collagen is often made from animal skins and chicken feet. It can suffocate the skin.*
- *Formaldehyde: found in cosmetics and nail-care products. It is an irritant and a carcinogen.*
- *Propylene glycol: found in skin and hair products. It is also used in brake fluid and antifreeze!*
- *Sodium lauryl sulphate: found in cosmetics, shampoos, toothpaste and cleaners. It is also used in garage-floor cleaners and engine degreasers, and is known in the scientific community as a skin irritant, absorbed and retained in the eyes, brain, heart and liver where it has a degenerative effect on cell membranes.*

## Emotional Agers

I have included 'emotional agers' (see list on page 9) because they all cause stress. And stress, as we've seen, is considered a toxin because it is one of the biggest causes of ageing, poor health and so many of those little, niggling problems we all suffer from as we get older. Recent research has revealed that stress shrinks the hippocampus, the main area for memory in the brain. And, as you'll read in the next chapter, a healthy stress-free brain means healthier hormones can be produced.

The Super Life chapter will certainly help you decide what you can do about the emotional agers such as stress and the rest of the book will help you with everything else on the list. None of us can live a completely natural life breathing in pure air, living on pure food and water and surviving without electricity and other stimuli. But you will be able to arm your body with plenty of stress-busting exercises and techniques by the time you have finished reading.

The next step in alternative ageing is healthy hormones, without which we can't hope to age slowly and healthily. Healthy hormones need healthy glands and, as you will see, there is a lot we can do to keep our glands from ageing.

# 2.

# Super Hormones

The word hormone comes from the Greek meaning 'to excite'. Hormones 'excite' each and every one of your trillions of cells and more than thirty have been discovered to date. Unfortunately our hormone levels actually decrease as we age and this has a profound effect on how we look and feel. At forty plus, oestrogen and testosterone levels fall. At fifty plus, dehydroepiandrosterone (DHEA), an invaluable anti-ageing hormone, and progesterone levels drop and at sixty they *all* decrease, dramatically. The really bad news is that the two hormones associated with ill health and ageing – insulin and cortisol – actually increase with age. This can lead to insulin resistance, diabetes and a whole host of niggling health problems. But don't despair, everything in this book is geared to improving the function of each cell, each gland, each organ in your body and, therefore, all your hormones as well, so you can enjoy old age in rude health.

## The Brain

The most important place to start on our alternative ageing journey is in the brain. It's where 90 per cent of all hormones are produced and regulated. Hormones are the brain's messengers and it sends them all over the body to control our cells. If the brain isn't performing properly hormone production can suffer. Dr Eric Braverman, author of *The Edge Effect* and a leading expert on our little grey cells, likens the brain to the roof of a house. 'People look after their houses but neglect the roof,' he says. 'The body won't function well if the brain's health is neglected and, most importantly for those of us who constantly lose our keys or forget things, the brain won't function at its best in a decrepit frame.' A great example is Alzheimer's. Some anti-ageing doctors think this awful condition is like plaque of the brain (they call it plaque, but you can think of it as 'rusting'). In other words, if you have healthy arteries taking oxygenated, nutritious blood to the brain, rather than furred up ones, then many forms of dementia and other brain disorders may well be avoided.

You are at your intellectual peak between twenty and thirty but it doesn't have to be downhill after that. Good nutrition and a few lifestyle changes can improve 'the roof of your house' more than you can imagine. I'm going to talk a lot about free radicals and how they affect the ageing process and your health in this book. You need look no further than the brain to see how they can speed up its deterioration. Free radicals cause oxidation, a kind of rusting, inside the delicate tissues of the brain. Stress and toxicity, both ingested and environmental, can speed the rates at which our brains 'rust' and, of course, if you don't *use* your brain it becomes less efficient. The brain is like any other muscle in the body; if it isn't exercised regularly it will shrink and become mushy and slack. So before you rush off to a shop for the latest, expensive supplement that is supposed to boost brainpower read on and learn how to feed your brain and keep it active for the rest of your life.

There are plenty of brain energy foods in the Super Foods chapter and lots on how to keep your brain from ageing throughout the rest of the book, but here are a few things you can think about eliminating from your life to give your brain and the neurotrans-mitters and hormones it produces the best possible chance.

## BRAIN ENEMIES

- *Lead*
- *Cadmium in cigarette smoke*
- *Pesticides*
- *Aluminium in cooking utensils*
- *Tap water*
- *Violent films*
- *Loud music*

- *Electromagnetic fields: microwaves, TVs, computers, mobile phones*
- *Alcohol – one drink can destroy up to one million brain cells!*

TOP TIP FOR A HEALTHY BRAIN

*Ballroom dancing, salsa, flamenco, whatever you enjoy – get out and do it. Scientists have discovered that dancing, and in particular the tango, can reduce the risk of developing Alzheimer's by 75 per cent because of the mental effort required by the brain.*

## Endocrine System

Now for a quick journey around the endocrine system – the group of glands that manufacture and secrete hormones: the pituitary, hypothalamus, pineal, thyroid, parathyroids, thymus, adrenals, pancreas and ovaries.

Imagine the endocrine system as an orchestra made up of nine glands that secrete hormones, which control everything in your body from when you get hungry to when you go to sleep. If one member of the orchestra is out of tune it affects the whole performance and your body won't function at full capacity. You can't have healthy hormones if you don't have healthy glands; you can't have healthy glands if your cells are not in tip-top condition, and you can't have healthy, youthful cells if they are not fed properly. This is why diet and lifestyle play such an important part in having happy hormones.

### The Pituitary Gland

This is the master gland, the conductor of the orchestra. Look after this gland and all the other glands in your body will perform in harmony to help you beat the ageing process. The pituitary gland is responsible for producing growth hormones (GH); these decrease as we get older. From the ages of thirty to fifty the decline of GH causes muscles to shrink and fat to increase and, suddenly, those hideous ageing signs look back at you from the mirror: saggy skin, wrinkles and abdominal fat.

Here are three top tips to help your pituitary produce the 'youth' hormone, GH:

TOP TIPS FOR A HEALTHY PITUITARY GLAND

*Exercise: fifteen minutes exercise a day will help produce GH.*
*Sleep well: the pituitary gland secretes GH mainly at night and helps repair the body's tissues while you sleep.*
*Give up coffee: two cups of coffee a day will cause GH levels to decrease.*

## The Hypothalamus Gland

Found at the base of your brain, this gland is the composer for the orchestra and it communicates with the conductor, the pituitary gland. It can take over and control your whole body completely if you are in a situation of extreme pain or stress, such as childbirth. In the last couple of decades endocrinologists have pinpointed this gland as the one that decides when we get thirsty, how hot we should be and whether we sweat or not. The hypothalamus interfaces with all the other glands and, in particular, the thyroid, pituitary and pineal glands.

## The Pineal Gland

The pineal gland is like a bit player. Mainstream doctors do not consider it terribly significant. However, the Greeks thought it important enough to call it the seat of the soul, and Eastern mystics and yogis refer to it as the third eye. I happen to think it one of the most important glands to look after if you want to sleep well and stay youthful.

The pineal is a small gland shaped like a pinecone, hence its name. It is situated near the centre of the brain. It produces melatonin in response to light, something we are sadly lacking in the UK during the winter months. It receives light via the optic nerves, so it can tell every single cell in your body when to sleep and when to wake. It's the body's own biological clock. But melatonin levels decrease as we get older, and by sixty we produce half as much as we did in our twenties – no wonder we sleep so badly the older we get and suffer from seasonal affective disorder (SAD) every winter.

There are plenty of natural ways to increase the effectiveness of your pineal gland, including how to take light straight into every cell in your body using super oils (see page 80).

But first, let's address sleep. A bad night's sleep is one of the most common complaints from my older clients. Nearly half of those over fifty regularly complain about sleeping badly and by the age of sixty many more are on their way to the doctor to get some help. Getting enough deep sleep is critical for anti-ageing because your cells do their biggest repair job while you are asleep. We need, on average, seven to eight hours' sleep a night, but not too much more.

Your new anti-ageing diet and lifestyle should certainly help you have a healthier pineal gland and get a decent night's sleep in no time. By the time you have reached the end of the book, you should be sleeping like a baby.

And here's a final, but slightly whacky, top tip given to me by a very serious medically trained doctor. He told me he had suffered a very bad night's sleep the preceding night because his hotel bed was facing the wrong way! For a good night's sleep, he said, the bed must face north, to match the planet's electromagnetic field.

 TOP TIP

*Lie with your feet towards north. This aligns your body with the electromagnetic field of the planet bringing your energies into harmony with the Earth.*

I have since seen this tip elsewhere and I must admit I usually find myself diagonally spread across the bed in the morning with my heels pointing north even though the only place for my bed is facing west!

TOP TIP FOR A HEALTHY PINEAL GLAND

*Ban the bedroom phone. A cordless phone base station interrupts melatonin production because of electro-magnetic radiation. Move any electrical equipment away from your bed.*

## The Thyroid Gland

The thyroid gland is shaped like a little bow tie and lies at the base of the throat. It only weighs about 30g but is absolutely crucial for the health of your body, your bones and for controlling your weight. It works much like a thermostat, making you feel hot or cold. Two of the more important hormones produced by the thyroid are thyroxine, which governs your metabolism, and calcitonin, which balances calcium levels in the blood and bones. The thyroid is important in the fight against ageing because it also promotes cell growth, hormone production and waste elimination. It is also the gland most likely to start malfunctioning whatever your age.

The World Health Organisation estimates that one to one and a half billion people are at risk from an under-active thyroid which is described by Dr Georges Mouton, a leading thyroid specialist, as the body running on 200 instead of 220 volts. One of the major signs of an under-active thyroid is suffering from freezing hands and feet, even if you are tucked up in a nice warm bed. Below are some of the many other symptoms. Please note these could be caused by other factors, so don't assume you have an under-active thyroid if you have, for example, brittle nails. On page 35 is a simple accurate test, the Barnes Axial Temperature Test, you can do yourself at home to find out for sure.

### SYMPTOMS OF AN UNDER-ACTIVE THYROID

- *Arthritis*
- *Brittle nails*
- *Cold extremities*
- *Constipation* ·

- *Depression*
- *Fluid retention*
- *Headaches*
- *Lack of concentration*
- *Lethargy*
- *Morning fatigue*
- *Muscle cramps*
- *Sudden weight gain*
- *Tinnitus*
- *Vertigo*

Dr Charles Heard is a scientist at the Welsh School of Pharmacy at Cardiff University with a special interest in the thyroid/iodine link. He believes that until now the importance of iodine in the diet for people with a thyroid condition has been overlooked. 'More and more clinical and anecdotal evidence points to the fact that a lack of iodine may be a contributory factor in thyroid dysfunction,' he says. There will be plenty of iodine-rich foods for you to eat in the Super Foods section on page 50, and plenty of other tips throughout the book to keep your thyroid healthy.

Some thyroid specialists think that eating less offal may be partly to blame for today's epidemic of under-active thyroids. Long before the days of mad cow disease, in the thrifty fifties, we ate liver or kidneys at least once a week. There may be something in this theory. Nowadays, many health practitioners prescribe animal glandulars (extracts taken from bovine glands) for clients suffering from thyroid dysfunction so why not eat them in the first place if you like them? I occasionally crave calf's liver, and when I do, I listen to my body and have it – usually with mashed potato and onions!

There are many other factors that can cause thyroid weakness. Here are a few:

## THYROID WEAKENERS

- *Heavy metals*
- *Environmental toxins*
- *Excess oestrogen*

- *Candida albicans*
- *Tonsillectomy*
- *Glandular fever*
- *Autoimmune disease*
- *Major surgery*
- *Excess iron*
- *Pregnancy*
- *Stress*
- *Chronic illness*
- *Severe dieting*
- *Insufficient protein*

Before you rush off to the doctor to check your thyroid you could do this very simple but accurate test. It was first described in the *Lancet* in 1945 and many thyroid specialists now consider it to be more accurate than a blood test.

### The Barnes Axial Temperature Test

The most accurate measurement of thyroid activity is the body's basal (resting) temperature which reflects your metabolic rate. Your thyroid sets the metabolic rate, so if your thyroid function is low, your basal temperature will be as well.

All you need is a mercury thermometer to measure your armpit temperature. Before you go to sleep, shake the thermometer and leave it by the bed. On waking, before doing anything else, place it in your armpit and wait a full 10 minutes. Record the temperature. Repeat for at least four days to obtain an average.

Men and post-menopausal women can take their temperature on any day, as long as they are not running a temperature. Women who are still menstruating will have fluctuating temperatures because of their hormonal cycles, so it is advisable to do this test on the second, third, fourth and fifth day of your period.

- *36.8–36.3 is normal*
- *36.3–36.0 is slightly low*
- *36.0–35.5 is low*
- *Less than 35.5 is very low*

If your temperature is low run your eyes over the list of iodine-suppressing foods and make sure you are not having any of them in excess – even those that are good for your health may be inhibiting your thyroid's ability to absorb iodine.

## IODINE SUPPRESSORS

- *Peanuts*
- *Cabbage*
- *Brussels sprouts*
- *Broccoli*
- *Kale*
- *Cauliflower*
- *Millet*
- *Soya products*

If you don't eat a lot of any of these foods, there is still some good news. Dr Mouton believes 77 per cent of people with a low functioning thyroid don't necessarily need medication. You can improve your thyroid's health by eating more iodine-rich foods such as deep-sea fish, cod or haddock for example, or sea vegetables as listed in Super Foods on page 75. There are also some very safe, natural supplements you can take, the main one being kelp. This is rich in iodine, and perfectly safe to take unless you are already taking thyroxine or a similar prescription drug. Apart from glandulars there are other supplements for the thyroid, but you will need to see a health practitioner or a doctor for these. Initially, try an iodine-rich diet for at least a month and then take your temperature again to see if it has risen.

TOP TIP

*Stop drinking tap water. Thyroid specialists are convinced the fluoride in it may be partly responsible for the epidemic of under-functioning thyroids. They say that fluoride can block the release of thyroxine.*

## The Parathyroid Glands

These are very close to the thyroid but have little connection to it. Two are just above the thyroid and two just below. They are very small and mustard yellow in colour. They were first discovered in 1925. Medical students were taught to associate them with moans, groans and stones. Their main role in life is to control the calcium level of the bloodstream within quite a narrow range. If the parathyroids are malfunctioning you can feel unwell, sleep badly and become irritable (moans), have a tendency to ulcers and pancreatitis (groans) and often produce kidney stones because of the high levels of calcium passing through them (stones). Fortunately, under-functioning parathyroids are very rare.

## Thymus

The thymus is found behind the sternum partly in the thorax and partly in the neck. It is critical to your health. I find it easy to remember what it does by thinking of T for T cells and T is for thymus. T cells are the ones that go into battle with infection and disease. The trouble is, the thymus is at its largest around puberty and then begins to atrophy until, in advanced age, it is replaced by fat. Most ageing diseases are caused by a much weakened immune system so it is paramount that we must do all we can to strengthen our immunity to help us stay healthy – and young.

There are plenty of examples of immune suppressors in the chapter on Super Agers, but the two biggest ones to discuss here are sugar and stress.

*Sugar*

In a recent study, youngsters with nice, big, healthy thymuses were given a cola drink that contained more than 60g of sugar. In just 45 minutes, their immune cells' ability to destroy infection had dropped by *half*!

*Stress*

It is well known by anyone working in the psycho-neuro-immunology field (which investigates the bridge between psychology and the nervous and immune systems) that stress is the number-one immune suppressor. But what may surprise you is that while prolonged stress weakens the immune system, big time, *short* bursts of an adrenaline rush have been found to *increase* the T-cell count. In fact, one lecturer told us that if everyone did a *weekly* parachute jump there would be no such thing as cancer! One jump in an entire lifetime is enough for me, but there are other, safer ways you can get regular thrills and have fun with your children or grandchildren at the same time.

TOP TIP: SUPPORT YOUR THYMUS

> *Have a weekly thrill: go to a fairground, whizz down a water slide, try a bungee jump, go roller blading, skiing. Try anything that gives you a short adrenaline rush. Your thymus will thank you for it, and it will keep you young!*

## The Adrenal Glands

The adrenal glands are little hat-shaped glands sitting on top of the kidneys and they play a really major role in anti-ageing.

During the menopause it is crucial that they work efficiently and don't become exhausted, because they have a lot of extra work to do. When the ovaries stop producing oestrogen, the adrenal glands take over and can help maintain oestrogen production at a level at which menopausal symptoms are kept at bay.

Their main function, though, is to produce cortisol in response to stress which stimulates our fight or flight mechanism and produces adrenaline so we can fight sabre-toothed tigers or run for our life. The trouble is we are constantly putting the body into fight or flight because we overload it with salt, sugar, alcohol, coffee and stress. This, eventually, over-stimulates the adrenal glands and they become too exhausted to produce any more adrenaline.

But by the time we get to seventy, cortisol levels soar, whether we are living on a diet of coffee and sugar or not. Cortisol can cause brain cells to die and excessive amounts can also weaken the immune system, decrease muscle mass and cause ageing skin. When cortisol increases, blood-sugar levels also increase and this can result in insulin resistance which accelerates ageing and fat storage.

If all this wasn't enough, between thirty and sixty the adrenals' secretion of DHEA, another invaluable anti-ageing hormone, declines. It is known as the 'mother of hormones' because it is converted into fifty other essential hormones, including oestrogens. By the time we are forty, we are producing half the amount we produced at thirty and by sixty-five DHEA levels can be reduced by 90 per cent.

Improved DHEA levels reduce body fat, improve skin texture, moisture and tone, increase sex drive and improve immunity, memory and bone density. It keeps weight down, and helps people look younger. But DHEA supplements are expensive and not available in the UK unless you see a specialist anti-ageing doctor.

However, there are two very natural and free ways to increase DHEA levels. One is meditation. People over forty-five who meditate have up to 47 per cent more DHEA, completely independent of diet, exercise, weight and alcohol consumption. You will find more on meditation and how to do it in the section on Super Life on page 202.

And the other that you may well not want to know about is urine therapy – drinking just a few drops of your pee! Yes, that got your attention. I know 99.9% of you will switch right off at this point, but it is worth researching, if you are not too horrified. DHEA is found in large quantities in your urine (as well as uric acid which has been found to destroy free radicals). Urine therapy is used, allegedly, by a whole host of famous people to keep them slim and looking remarkably younger than their counterparts. But it does have to be caffeine-, nicotine-, alcohol- and fish-free urine! If you drink 2 litres of water a day, and eat a mostly vegetarian diet, your urine will be without smell, taste or colour. As an aside, most beauty products contain cow or horse's uric acid which you put on your face quite happily every day! I have tried urine therapy but can't go on a proper regime till I have given up my daily cup of coffee – which I can't cope with until I have finished this book!

Finally, adrenal insufficiency is also linked to an under-functioning thyroid so specialists often treat the adrenals first. There will be details of adrenal supporting foods in Super Foods, but first you may want to check this list and see if you may be suffering from adrenal insufficiency.

### SIGNS OF ADRENAL INSUFFICIENCY

- *Prolonged stress*
- *Chronic fatigue*
- *Lower back and loin pain*
- *Poor exercise tolerance*
- *Hissing in the ears*
- *Salt craving*
- *Dark rings under the eyes*
- *Loss of body hair*
- *Dry, thin skin.*

Saliva and urine tests are more accurate than blood tests if you feel you need to be tested by a doctor, but rest assured that if you follow the suggestions in Super Agers (page 7) and give up salt, sugar, alcohol, coffee and stress you will be well on the way to having stronger adrenal glands.

## Pancreas

The pancreas is a greyish-pink gland about 12–15cm long, sitting behind the stomach with its tail touching the spleen and its head tucked into the duodenum, shaped like a fish! Its main job is to secrete the hormones insulin and glucagon, which both affect carbohydrate metabolism. This is the gland to really look after if you want to stay slim, energetic and healthy.

When you eat sugar or a sugary carbohydrate such as a baked potato, the pancreas releases insulin to control the sudden rise in blood-sugar levels. Half an hour later, you'll crave more sugar to repeat the blood-sugar high. So the roller-coaster ride of extreme blood-sugar highs followed by blood-sugar lows begins. Stress, forgetting to eat and living on stimulants such as sugar, nicotine, caffeine and alcohol can all contribute to high blood-sugar levels. Every time we have that extra cup of coffee or second chocolate bar, the level of glucose in the blood surges and so do our energy levels – temporarily. This can lead to headaches, irritability, mood swings, low energy, feeling cold and, eventually, chronic insulin exhaustion or insulin resistance because the pancreas is being asked to produce insulin so often it just runs out. Result? Diabetes and heart disease.

Our twenty-first century diet with foods high in sugar, stimulants and refined carbohydrates, has led to an epidemic of blood-sugar problems: insulin resistance, obesity and adult-onset diabetes particularly, but not solely, among the baby boomers. We've all turned into carb and sugar junkies and our health is suffering because of it.

### SIGNS OF INSULIN RESISTANCE

- *Needing to constantly nibble between meals*
- *Needing a cigarette to get going*
- *Bingeing on things you crave*
- *Gobbling food down*
- *Needing a coffee in the morning to get going*
- *Desperate for a chocolate bar at teatime*

- *Starving by supper*
- *Craving alcohol every evening*
- *Can't live without bread, potatoes or bananas*
- *Sensitive to light*

If you think you may be suffering from the blood-sugar blues or are on your way to a pre-diabetic state, you will find the perfect eating plan in the form of the Glycaemic Index diet on page 114 in the Super Anti-Ageing Diet section. For example, seemingly healthy food such as mashed potato is very high on the glycaemic index (GI) and can release sugar into the bloodstream almost as fast as sweets or chocolate. But grains such as brown basmati rice are much lower on the scale and release sugar slowly so that energy is sustained over a much longer time and blood-sugar highs and lows become a thing of the past.

 TOP TIP

*If you hit the afternoon teatime dip and get a craving for a huge bar of chocolate, drink a pint of water at body temperature instead. There is nothing that evens out blood-sugar fluctuations quicker than this.*

## The Ovaries

Finally, two little glands that cause us the most obvious and annoying problems throughout women's lives, as well as being essential for reproduction. The ovaries are a pair of glands, as I'm sure you know, that secrete oestrogen and progesterone, responsible for: pregnancy, periods, mood swings, acne and the menopause.

The first hormonal changes that lead to the menopause can start in the thirties, but more usually in the early forties, and can last for ten to fifteen years. This is when oestrogen levels are on the decline. Once over fifty, there is a dramatic decline in progesterone and testosterone production as well. Eventually periods cease, and you are considered to be menopausal when it has been at least six months since the last period.

However, some women have an imbalance of hormones all through their menstruating life, so below are listed a few symptoms to look out for, oh joy! Should you think you are deficient in one hormone or another there are plenty of foods that supply natural progesterone or oestrogen suggested in the book. There are also suggestions for relieving the worst symptoms of fluctuating hormones – whether you are menopausal, perimenopausal or still menstruating.

As this book is aimed at baby boomers there isn't specific advice on period problems such as PMT, headaches or painful breasts in this chapter, though an increase in your consumption of omega-3-rich oils recommended on page 78 will certainly help. But there is a great deal of information in the rest of the book that will benefit you, at whatever stage of your menstruating life you are, and I'm sure symptoms such as bloating or PMT will disappear once you have tried a few of the suggestions.

## SYMPTOMS OF PROGESTERONE DEFICIENCY

- *PMT*
- *Fluid retention*
- *Sweats*
- *Osteoporosis*
- *Fibroids*
- *Heavy periods*

## SYMPTOMS OF OESTROGEN DOMINANCE

- *Weight gain*
- *Fluid retention*
- *Painful breasts*
- *PMT*
- *Heavy periods*
- *Fibroids*

I should add that some of the symptoms on these lists may have other causes so always *see your doctor* for a proper diagnosis.

## SYMPTOMS OF PERIMENOPAUSE

- *Irregular periods*
- *Acne*
- *Weight gain*
- *Hot flushes*
- *Irritability*
- *Depression*
- *Forgetfulness*

The time leading up to the menopause, the perimenopause, is often characterized by irregular periods and changes such as shorter or longer, lighter or heavier bleeding. It can start as early as thirty-five and last ten to fifteen years. I knew I was perimenopausal when I started getting spots, for the first time in my life, all over my chin and a very helpful assistant in a well-known high-street chemist shouted across the shop that it was probably my hormones!

The menopause is a time when oestrogen and progesterone decline to a point where menstruation stops completely. This is a completely natural point in women's lives. The average age for the menopause in the UK is fifty. The good news is that many of the symptoms can be completely avoided if, like me, you make some simple changes to lifestyle and diet.

## SYMPTOMS OF OESTROGEN DEFICIENCY

- *Loss of skin elasticity*
- *Wrinkles around the mouth*
- *Palpitations*
- *Disturbed sleep*
- *Loss of libido*
- *Vaginal dryness*

Don't forget that the adrenal glands can replace up to 75 per cent of the oestrogen levels found pre-menopause, so they need to be well looked after and fed with the highest-octane fuel to keep them functioning at their most efficient to allow you to sail through the menopause – if you haven't already done so.

Some women are, unfortunately, more likely to be at risk of menopausal symptoms than others, so these women need to consider the more orthodox route to sailing through the menopause:

## WOMEN MORE AT RISK

- *Underweight women*
- *Had a hysterectomy*
- *Had radiotherapy*
- *Had chemotherapy*
- *Smokers*

Only 10 per cent of menopausal women in the UK have symptoms considered severe enough to warrant Hormone Replacement Therapy (HRT). This is artificially synthesized oestrogen, derived from horses' urine, which 'fools' the body into believing it is not menopausal, much like the Pill 'fools' the body into believing it's pregnant. The trouble is, apart from the health scares, when HRT is stopped, the menopausal symptoms usually return more severely and dramatically. I have always been told that HRT is a bit like using a steamroller to crush a nut so, unless there is no other way of dealing with the menopause, I would rather take the natural prevention route.

There are masses of natural alternatives suggested throughout the book, the safest and easiest being to eat foods high in phytoestrogens (see page 71): natural plant chemicals that bind to oestrogen-receptor cells in the body and mimic the hormone safely. But first, a quick 'how to help' those ghastly symptoms from your fluctuating hormones.

DO NOT TAKE ANY OF THE HERBS MENTIONED IF YOU ARE ALREADY ON HRT OR HAVE A HISTORY OF BREAST CANCER. ALWAYS SEE AN EXPERT FIRST.

*Hot Flushes*
These are often related to fluctuating blood-sugar levels as well as fluctuating hormones, so avoid sugar and drink 2 litres of water a

day. Avoid smoking, drinking alcohol and coffee, they all exacerbate hot flushes as do spicy and processed foods. Make sure you follow the tips in the section on Super Bowels on page 153, to avoid a toxic build-up which can also aggravate symptoms.

The herbs black cohosh and sage have both been found to reduce hot flushes dramatically by as much as 50 per cent. They contain phytoestrogens which are plant forms of oestrogen and bind to hormone receptors. They act as adaptogens lowering high oestrogen levels or boosting low ones. They also help rebalance the hypothalamus and regulate sweat production.

### Loss of Libido

The foods in the Super Foods chapter will help enormously because many contain a natural form of progesterone which helps a flagging libido.

### Stress and Depression

Low progesterone levels and a deficiency of B vitamins and magnesium can cause irritability and moodiness. You will get plenty of foods rich in these three essentials in the Super Foods chapter.

If you feel very depressed, there are herbs such as St John's Wort or lemon balm. But a really safe option are the wolfberries mentioned in Super Supplements (see page 129) – more of a happy berry than a supplement!

Get plenty of regular exercise to encourage the body's natural production of happy chemicals – endorphins. There's much more on the whys and wherefores of exercise in the Super Fit chapter.

### Osteoporosis

Research has shown that onset of brittle bones during the menopause can be due to nutritional deficiencies, especially during teenage years when the bones are still growing, as well as a drop in oestrogen levels. It is worth noting that more and more youngsters in their twenties have bone-density results comparable to people thirty years their senior. The reason? They have lived on a diet of fizzy drinks which, whether they are low-cal or full sugar, are loaded with phosphorus which drags calcium out of the bones. Thin, meat-eating women who eat high-protein, high-salt diets are also most prone to osteoporosis. Too much protein in the diet leaches calcium out of the bones.

There is plenty of advice on how to avoid osteoporosis, and even reverse it, later in the book (see page 148). You may want to consider reducing your intake of red meat, salt, cigarettes, soft drinks and alcohol and increasing the amount of exercise you take.

HRT can protect you against osteoporosis, but as soon as you stop taking it bone density falls very quickly. Improving your diet and lifestyle *now* is a far better long-term solution. You may wonder why I haven't mentioned calcium. Calcium is essential for strong bones, but magnesium is equally essential because calcium cannot be absorbed properly without it. Anyone on a calcium supplement should make sure it has equal amounts of magnesium. Not many doctors seem aware of this. As far as calcium-packed foods go, there are loads for you to choose from in the Super Foods and Super Supplements chapters and plenty of advice on how to strengthen your bones in the Super Fit chapter (see pages 50, 126 and 182).

TOP TIP

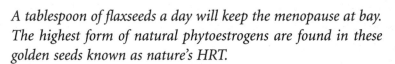

*A tablespoon of flaxseeds a day will keep the menopause at bay. The highest form of natural phytoestrogens are found in these golden seeds known as nature's HRT.*

### Fatigue
This can be caused by night sweats, insomnia, anxiety or anaemia due to heavy periods, as well as nutritional deficiencies.

### Aches and Pains
A build-up of uric acid as well as low oestrogen levels can cause joint pain. The Anti-Ageing Diet emphasizes alkaline rather than acidic foods so follow the Raw and Living diet on page 109 as much as possible if you are suffering from aching joints. Nettle tea can also help dissolve uric acid in the joints.

*Bladder Problems*
This will be covered in full in the Super Bod chapter but you may want to know why everything goes pear-shaped in that region when we hit the menopause. Low levels of oestrogen can cause a thinning of the lining of the bladder which may lead to mild incontinence.

For a more stable bladder:

AVOID

---

- *Coffee*
- *Fizzy drinks*
- *Alcohol*
- *Sugar*
- *Fruit juice*

*Poor Skin and Nails*
Falling oestrogen levels can cause thinning hair and poor calcium absorption (usually caused by a lack of magnesium) and can make your nails brittle and cause your skin to lose its elasticity.

*Vaginal Dryness*
Caused by low oestrogen levels as well as a lack of essential fats and vitamin E. Don't use commercial soaps for cleaning that area and do use vitamin E internally as well as externally. There are also natural vaginal lubricants on the market should you need a little help.

My personal, all-round favourite for treating most menopausal symptoms is wild yam cream. The wild Mexican yam is the plant that led to the development of HRT and the Pill. It has a high concentration of diosgenin, which has a similar molecular structure to progesterone. The creams are easily absorbed through the skin, but you can also buy supplements, tinctures and gels for conditions such as vaginal dryness. Be careful where you buy wild yam, because most are just ground-up root. What you want to buy is a wild yam extract that has been 'pharmaceutically standardized in its extraction', see Resources on page 235.

So there it is, a journey round the endocrine system and all those glands that keep you ticking over but are maybe not working as well as they could be. If you want to know more on how to get the best out of your glands, there is a great series of exercises in Super Fit especially for the endocrine system on page 195.

I'm sure by now you realize what foods and liquids need to be eliminated for the sake of healthy glands, as they crop up over and over again. Now let's see which foods you need to incorporate for the sake of ageing well and healthily.

# 3.

# Super Foods

As you have probably gathered by now, if you want to live long, look young and stay healthy, you need healthy cells. One of the reasons we age appears to be the accumulation of toxins and free radicals that cause glycation and oxidation. Free radicals damage the cells, wound your DNA and 'rust' your cells. However, if we eat plenty of antioxidants as well as other age-defying nutrients, we can counter the damage free radicals and oxidation cause.

Here's a list of the anti-ageing warriors your body needs, and why. This will be followed by recommended Super Foods that will provide you with those anti-ageing warriors and plenty more.

CAROTENOIDS slow the ageing process and help protect against cancer.

FLAVONOIDS are twenty times more potent than vitamin C and fifty times stronger than vitamin E. They protect your skin and increase immunity against disease.

VITAMIN A and BETA-CAROTENE give you supple, firm, unlined skin. They promote collagen and elastin production and strengthen your eyesight.

VITAMIN C is well known for reducing the duration of colds or flu. It is also essential for guarding your brain and eyes against oxidation as well as repairing skin damage caused by the sun, pollution or smoking.

VITAMIN E is superb for skin and tissue repair, as well as preventing cell oxidation and destroying free radicals.

VITAMIN D helps your bones absorb and use calcium and magnesium.

GLYCONUTRIENTS can awaken the immune system as if from a coma! They are not antioxidants as such but they do generate the potent antioxidants that keep the body young.

B VITAMINS are one of the most important anti-agers. A full range of B vitamins are essential for older people because they act like the catalytic spark plugs of the body strengthening your nervous system, mental health and digestion.

MINERALS such as magnesium, potassium, sodium and calcium are essential for optimum cell health but are the ones most likely to be out of balance. The natural place for sodium and calcium is *outside* the cell while magnesium and potassium should be *inside* the cell. Anything that changes that polarity can cause stress at a cellular level and stop the cells doing their job keeping you healthy and young. The trouble with our twenty-first-century diet is that we consume an abundance of calcium and sodium but are seriously deficient in magnesium and potassium. That means the electrolyte balance is disrupted, the cells don't function or cleanse properly and you haven't a hope in hell of fighting ageing.

> **95 per cent of us are seriously depleted in potassium**
> **75 per cent of us are seriously depleted in magnesium**

All four minerals are needed in perfect balance if you want a healthy heart, hormones and bones.

SILICA AND SULPHUR for collagen renewal and preventing sagging skin and wrinkles.

ZINC AND SELENIUM for strengthening the immune system. They are also essential for glutathione and superoxide dismutase (SOD) synthesis: two unpronounceable words that mean your body is protected against free-radical damage and oxidation!

IODINE for supporting the thyroid and controlling metabolism.

CHROMIUM for regulating blood-sugar levels.

IRON for producing strong blood cells and protecting the DNA from malfunctioning.

FIBRE without which your digestion will be sluggish causing tired-looking skin.

ESSENTIAL FATS in the form of omega-3 and 6. There is plenty of omega-6 available in everyone's diet but, unless you eat oily fish four times a week, most people are deficient in omega-3, which is needed, quite simply, by every single cell in your body for:

> brain health
> heart health
> skin health
> joint health
> reducing inflammation
> improving digestion
> boosting metabolism
> reducing depression
> hormone production

Wherever and whenever possible I always recommend buying the freshest and purest fruit and vegetables you can afford – within reason. But before you fill your basket with organic produce, first look at the labels and see how far it has travelled. In an ideal world, food should be grown locally and you should eat it in season. I don't see the point of buying organic apples if they have been flown all the way from New Zealand, or Spanish strawberries that have been ripening en route for three days, when the UK produces some of the best apples and strawberries in the world. The longer it takes from farm to fork, the fewer nutrients will be available by the time you eat that apple or strawberry. But any fruit or vegetable you juice, blend or purée needs to be as free of chemicals as possible. If you are juicing a fresh, whole carrot you are not only extracting 90 per cent of its vitamins and minerals but also 90 per cent of any pesticides.

The compromise, for the sake of your health and your purse, may lie in the growing number of farmers' markets and home-delivery schemes. You can buy direct from local farmers knowing the food has been grown within a thirty-mile radius of where you live. Even in cities. The fruit and veg will be more nutrient rich because it hasn't been ripened artificially during a long journey. It will be cheaper because the growers have cut out the middleman and more environmentally friendly because it has used less food miles. It will also be seasonal so you will be eating what you were genetically meant to eat at that time of the year.

## Super Veg

The word vegetable comes from the Latin meaning 'to enliven or animate'. So if we want to be lively, animated and youthful we need to eat our veg!

Vegetables are full of immune-boosting, disease-fighting vitamins and minerals such as vitamins A and C, folic acid (from the word foliage), beta-carotene and selenium. The greener the vegetables the richer in nutrients. Cruciferous vegetables, plants that grow in the shape of a cross, such as broccoli, Brussels sprouts, cabbage, kale, mustard, horseradish and cauliflower, have been found to be rich in anti-cancer properties (ally1-isothiocyanate) and glucosinolates – nutrients that help the liver detox and strengthen. But don't forget these vegetables are also to be avoided in huge quantities if you suffer from an under-active thyroid. If you have been diagnosed with an under-active thyroid, check with your doctor how much is too much. According to the thyroid specialist Dr Georges Mouton, swede and rape are also possible thyroid disruptors, because they contain goitrine.

A quick word about sprouts of all kinds. I used to hate things like alfalfa sprouts, but have grown to love them and now add them to my salads whenever I can. They are a top anti-ageing food because they are so full of nutrients. They contain chlorophyll, silica, beta-carotene, bioflavonoids, B vitamins, amino acids and minerals. They are also 'living' so you take into your body all the energy, goodness and power that enables them to grow from tiny seeds into a strong, fully grown plant. If you want youthful cells, eat your sprouts.

If you can't find them in the shops, they are really easy to grow at home. You just need a sprouting jar and some seeds.

## REASONS TO EAT SUPER VEG

- *Four times more potassium and magnesium than sodium and calcium, so the right proportions for cell health*
- *Low-fat food*
- *80 per cent water*
- *A good balance of carbohydrate and protein*
- *High fibre for healthy bowels*

Here's a list of the top anti-ageing vegetables that you should eat regularly. A really good buy are the salad bags you can get in all supermarkets, containing rocket, watercress and spinach giving you a mineral-rich, raw salad that provides your body with everything it needs in the mineral department to keep you young.

Marrows, tomatoes, peppers and avocado are, strictly speaking, fruits as they contain their seeds, but for the sake of simplicity you will find them all under vegetables.

## Vegetable Shopping List

Alfalfa sprouts: 'father' of all foods, a top anti-ageing veg
Artichoke: shifts toxins, clears the skin and is a blood-sugar stabilizer
Asparagus: a natural diuretic and high in protein
Aubergine: contains anthocyanins, which are potent antioxidants
Avocado: my favourite food, high in antioxidants, especially vitamin E, B, potassium and lipase, a fat-busting enzyme. Not fattening, as it is always eaten raw and raw food does NOT put on weight. It is a top anti-ageing food
Bean sprouts: a 'living' food, therefore anti-ageing
Beetroot: detoxifies the liver and gall bladder and cleans the colon
Broccoli: rich in glucosinolates, helps the liver to detox
Brussels sprouts: rich in glucosinolates, helps the liver to detox
Cabbage: rich in glucosinolates and selenium, protects the immune system

Carrots: one single carrot contains 7 different active anti-cancer compounds as well as enough beta-carotene for one day. Protects against ultraviolet radiation and is a fantastic liver tonic. High in glyconutrients and selenium to boost the immune system

Cauliflower: rich in glucosinolates, helps the liver detox and is high in vitamin C

Celery: high in natural sodium and a natural diuretic

Chicory: stimulates the liver

Corn: vitamin C

Courgettes: folic acid, potassium and vitamins A and C

Cucumber: rich in silicon and sulphur for strong skin, nails and hair

Dandelion leaves: rich in all anti-ageing minerals

Dark green lettuce: all the main anti-ageing minerals

Dill: an anti-bloater

Endive: contains potassium and iron

Fennel: shifts toxins and clears the skin. A liver and digestion stimulant. It contains oestragole, an oestrogen-like compound

Green beans: vitamin K, essential for blood clotting and strong bones

Kale: rich in glucosinolates to help the liver detox

Leeks: high in glyconutrients

Lettuce: high in silicon, which supports your skin

Mushrooms: see SUPER FUNGI, they really are super! (Unless you suffer from arthritis or candida). High in chromium and selenium

Mustard greens: high in glucosinolates and vitamins A, C and E

Nettles: high in iron and all essential minerals

Olives: high in vitamin E for young, healthy skin

Onions: shifts toxins and clears the skin and is high in glyconutrients. Raw red ones are best. Rich in quercetin bioflavonoids which protect the cells from free radicals. High in chromium

Parsley: a great adrenal supporter, rich in iron

Parsnips: high in beta-carotene, the more orange the more they have

Peas: high in galactose, which acts as a free-radical scavenger

Peppers: don't eat raw green peppers, they are unripe and hard on

the digestion. Red, yellow and orange peppers are beta-carotene
rich

Radishes: high in glyconutrients

Spinach: high in folic acid and iron

Spring onions: high in potassium, calcium, magnesium and vitamin A

Squashes: high in vitamin A, C and potassium

Swiss chard: high in magnesium, vitamins C, A and K

Sweet potatoes: always pick deep-orange-coloured ones for
maximum nutrients. High in beta-carotene

Tomatoes: high in bioflavonoids and lycopene, anti-cancer, and
high in galactose which acts as a free-radical scavenger

Watercress: rich in vitamin C and glucosinolates that help the liver
detox. Also good for the adrenal glands

## Super Fungi

Mushrooms, especially Japanese ones, are high in glyconutrients
that support the body's ability to neutralize oxidative damage.
They help the body fight off pathogens but take time to work,
from a month to six weeks. Some of them are so potent they are
considered approved drugs in Japan for their ability to encourage
the body to produce stronger T cells.

Buy organic mushrooms and don't eat them raw, as the glyconutrients stay trapped if they are not cooked. Dried mushrooms are
better than fresh, if they haven't been grown locally.

### Fungi Shopping List

Shiitake: increases immunity, is anti-viral and helps relieve chronic
fatigue

Cordyceps: reduces stress, strengthens bones and reduces cholesterol

Maitake: helps with weight loss, reduces blood-sugar levels and
increases immunity

Reishi: can help relieve insomnia, and increase immunity, energy
  levels and longevity
Oyster: helps to absorb fat and increase immunity

## MUSHROOM TEA

Place your chosen mushrooms in a pot and add water to cover.
Bring to a gentle boil and then reduce to a simmer. Cover and
cook until the mushrooms are tender. Drink the broth.

## Super Fruit

Fruit is one of nature's perfect foods: natural, healthy, juicy and,
like us, largely made up of water. Fruit is also quite clever because
it carries the seeds for the next generation within it, which makes
it extremely nutrient-rich. I still haven't quite worked out why
strawberries are the only fruit with their seeds on the outside, but
they are higher in vitamin C, pound for pound, than oranges. All
fruit is essential for anti-ageing.

All berries are extremely high in antioxidants so are the TOP
FRUIT when it comes to any anti-ageing diet. They are also
high in lutein and zeaxanthin, plant chemicals that help maintain
healthy eyes.

### REASONS TO EAT SUPER FRUIT

- *Life-bearing food*
- *70–90 per cent water content*
- *25–55 per cent healthy sugars*
- *High in potassium, magnesium, calcium and sodium*
- *Rich in the anti-ageing vitamins A, C, Bs and E*
- *Low in fat*
- *High in fibre*

## Fruit Shopping List

Apples: one a day keeps the doctor away. High in chromium, boron and vitamin C

Apricots: rich in potassium and vitamin A

Bananas: high in potassium and vitamin $B_6$

Blackberries: high in bioflavonoids and vitamin C

Blackcurrants: high in vitamin C, calcium and bioflavonoids

Blueberries: extremely high in antioxidants, fifty nutrients per berry

Cherries: high in bioflavonoids

Coconut: good adrenal supporter

Cranberries: high in vitamin C and contain one of the highest levels of phenols, a potent antioxidant

Figs: rich in potassium, calcium and galactose, a free-radical scavenger

Grapefruit (pink): high in vitamin C, prevents fluid retention and cleanses the liver

Grapes: high in selenium, boron for bones, galactose, a free-radical scavenger and resveratrol, an anti-oxidizer

Guavas: very high in vitamin C

Kiwis: flown an awfully long way! But high in vitamin C and contain a natural digestive enzyme

Lemons: very high in vitamin C and calcium. Make the system alkaline

Lime: very high vitamin C and makes the system alkaline

Mango: gut cleaner and contains a digestive enzyme

Melons: very high in magnesium and vitamin A

Nectarines: diuretic, cleansing and easily digested

Oranges: vitamin C and selenium and helps the liver to detox

Papaya: gut cleaner and digestive enzyme plus vitamin A, vitamin C and potassium

Peaches: diuretic, cleansing and easily digested

Pears: one of the few foods no one is allergic to. High in chromium, and has some boron

Pineapple: a gut cleaner and a natural digestive enzyme in the form of bromelaine

Pomegranates: rich in oestrone, a natural form of oestrogen

Strawberries: more vitamin C, pound for pound, than oranges
Tangerines: vitamin C and zinc and help liver detox
Watermelon: a natural diuretic and cleanser

Some fruits can be hard on the digestive system and can cause problems in people with sensitive digestive systems, Candida, or other health problems such as blood-sugar issues so don't eat any fruit in excess – no more than five portions a day.

## Dried Fruit

Dried fruit is a wonderful source of vitamins and minerals but is also extremely high in sugar, can encourage weight gain, harm your teeth and cause diarrhoea and flatulence if eaten in excess. Eat dried fruit in moderation – one or two pieces a day – and buy organic wherever possible.

## Dried Fruit Shopping List

Apricots: extremely high in potassium
Blueberries: rich in antioxidants
Cranberries: rich in antioxidants
Figs: more calcium than any other fruit
Raisins: high in magnesium and potassium

# Super Fish

According to many anti-ageing experts, if you want a firm, toned, young face and body, you need to eat a fresh supply of top-quality animal protein, preferably oily fish, every day. Protein is essential for cellular repair as the building blocks of our cells are composed of the amino acids found in animal proteins.

Although raw foodists and vegetarians would disagree (you can read much more about this in the Super Anti-Ageing Diet chapter and make up your own mind) without animal or fish protein our ageing process accelerates. Dermatologist Dr Nicholas Perricone claims that patients who start eating a diet rich in high-quality protein, such as salmon, five times a day, see their skin firm up and lift within weeks.

The best way to combine eating plenty of protein and those skin-plumping essential oils, is to eat oily fish regularly. It is more easily digested than red meat, lower in saturated fat, and is packed full of omega-3 essential fats, calcium, magnesium, selenium, zinc and iodine.

Omega-3 fatty acids help produce the prostaglandin 3 series (PG3) which has been shown to reduce the inflammation of arthritis, blood pressure and heart disease as well as improving cholesterol levels, hormone production, metabolism, nerve transmission and gut function. In fact everything! Especially plumped-up, young-looking skin.

Oily fish, especially salmon, also contains DMAE, a powerful antioxidant that stimulates nerve function and causes the muscles to contract and tighten under the skin.

If you don't fancy fish you can still reap the benefits from a daily dose of two 1000mg EPA fish-oil capsules, available in most health stores. There is a lot more about EPA fish oils in the Super Supplements chapter and there are plenty of omega-3 vegetarian options under seeds and nuts on page 69.

FISH-OIL NUTRIENTS

- *Vitamin A – healthy eyes*
- *Omega-3 – healthy heart, joints and brain*
- *Zinc – immune system*
- *DMAE – plumped-up skin*
- *Nucleotides – for healthy DNA*

## Fish Shopping List

Farmed fish, such as salmon, spend their lives in small, crowded pens where they are hand-fed pellets with added colourings. A wild salmon migrates thousands of miles through the open ocean, hunting its omega-3-rich plankton. This makes it leaner and more omega-3 rich, as well as more expensive.

If you are on a budget, the best and cheapest oily fish is tinned salmon from Alaska: the coldest, cleanest sea on the planet. I can't vouch for how nutrient-rich the fish were before being canned but at least they come from relatively toxin-free water. Tinned tuna is fine, in oil or spring water, not sodium-packed brine and tinned sardines pack more of a calcium punch than a pint of milk, if you eat the bones!

## OILY FISH IN ORDER OF OMEGA-3 CONTENT

- *Salmon*
- *Mackerel*
- *Albacore tuna (more common in the Mediterranean)*
- *Blue fin tuna (very scarce)*
- *Sardines*
- *Herring*
- *Anchovies (silver ones)*
- *Trout*
- *Atlantic halibut*
- *Yellow fin tuna*
- *Tinned tuna*

There are lots of other fish that contain omega-3, in smaller amounts, and many others that are low in this essential fat but high in other nutrients. Shellfish are an excellent source of protein, high in zinc and copper, and much easier to digest and lower in fat than meat. However, shellfish are also high in cholesterol and collect toxins, especially arsenic and mercury, as they love feeding around sewage pipes. So if you love shellfish, moderation is the key.

TOP TIP

*After a heart attack a person eating oily fish three times a week halves the risk of another.*

## Super Meats

There is a place for eating meat on an anti-ageing diet if you are used to eating it regularly, have a healthy digestion and no serious health problems. Oily fish would be much better for your skin's appearance and for the health of your heart, joints and brain, but some meats have health and anti-ageing benefits as well. In particular, an antioxidant called carnosine, found in lamb, poultry and wild game, protects the brain from free-radical damage and can slow down wrinkle formation.

So if you eat meat and two veg every Sunday, have no health problems and are not prepared to swap your joint of beef for fish, at least make it meat and *six* veg and choose a meat from the shopping list. If it's organic, free range or 'wild', it will be lower in saturated fat and a healthier alternative to bog-standard supermarket red-meat cuts.

Here's your shopping list in order of health benefits. This is meant for occasional consumption only and the lower down the list your favourite meat is, the more important it is that you buy organic, free-range and grass-fed produce wherever possible.

### Super Meat Shopping List

Game: pheasant, partridge, venison, rabbit, wild boar – iron levels are much higher than in any other meat, other than liver

Poultry: chicken, turkey – less fatty than most meats and easier to digest and assimilate

Goat

Bison

Buffalo

Offal: liver, kidneys – contain a very concentrated source of vitamins, especially B5, B12, minerals and DHA (docasal hexaenoic acid), the most effective of the omega-3 fatty acids, and are beneficial for thyroid health

Lamb: this is one of the few foods that cannot cause an allergy. It is more easily assimilated in the body than most other red meats and is less acidic.

Beef
Pork
Meat products

## Super Eggs

Eggs contain *half* the daily nutritional elements required by the brain, nerves and organs. They are regarded as providing the most complete protein available in a single source. Protein makes up half the egg, the rest is fat, two-thirds of which is unsaturated. Eggs are rich in lecithin, which helps reduce cholesterol not increase it. The dreaded cholesterol found in egg yolk is not the cause of raised cholesterol levels by itself, it is only when combined with a high saturated-fat diet that cholesterol levels zoom up i.e. the great British fried-egg sandwich is not going to help your arteries! Eggs also contain an amino acid called N-acetyl cysteine which helps produce the antioxidant compound glutathione that helps your liver detox.

Unless you have high cholesterol and have been told not to eat more than two eggs a week, have them often but don't fry them. Baby boomers will remember the 'Go to Work on an Egg' campaign, and I couldn't agree more. Whether boiled, poached or scrambled, eggs make an excellent breakfast giving you a slow release of energy throughout the day and giving your adrenals an important protein boost first thing.

## Super Soya or not so Super?

The soya bean is made up of saponins, amino acids, minerals and isoflavones, which belong to the family of phytoestrogens, well documented for helping maintain a healthy heart and bones, reducing menopausal symptoms and preventing breast cancer. It is now also well documented that large quantities of soya can *increase* the risk of breast cancer, because of the oestrogenic action isoflavones may have. Far from balancing hormone levels, the isoflavones and other toxic substances may disrupt the endocrine system leading to problems with infertility, thyroid disorders, early onset of puberty in children and a depletion of vital nutrients such as zinc, iodine and calcium.

I leave you to decide whether or not to include soya in your diet. I would just add that all foods have a potential for toxicity if they are over-consumed. If you love soya try and eat it in the fermented form of miso, tempeh and Tamari as the Japanese do. Miso, especially, is particularly good as it is rich in an alkaloid called dipicolinic acid, which helps drag toxins out of the body safely, as well as helping to produce healthy intestinal flora.

If you are worried about your phytoestrogen intake there is a much safer alternative – seeds (see page 71). For vegetarians, the next section on pulses will give you a healthier protein alternative to soya.

## Super Pulses

Unlike wheat, it seems we have been eating pulses for more than ten thousand years. Beans, peas and lentils contain compounds that can help protect you against cancer (inositol pentakisphosphate, if you must know!). Pulses also contain natural progesterone, for happy hormones, and they're high in nutrients and low in calories.

### REASONS TO EAT SUPER PULSES

- *High protein*
- *High fibre*
- *Low fat*
- *High anti-cancer compounds*
- *High in zinc, potassium, magnesium, calcium and iron*
- *High in folic acid*
- *Reduce homocysteine – an amino acid that encourages clogged arteries and heart disease*
- *Stabilize blood-sugar levels*

- *Contain saponins for increasing immunity and lowering cholesterol*

Although pulses are a good source of protein, they are an incomplete protein because they do not contain all eight essential amino acids, which make up proteins. To make them complete, they need to be eaten with grains. A good example is baked beans on toast, or hummus and brown rice.

One of the main problems with eating pulses is that they give you wind, caused by the oligosaccharides (sugars) in the beans fermenting away in the lower intestines. If the beans are soaked overnight and then rinsed you will get rid of most of that sugar. You can always get ready cooked canned pulses to save time and your gut.

## Super Dairy and Super Alternatives

For vegetarians and cheese lovers alike, this section advises you on the best of the dairy products and why it's OK to consume them in moderation along with some true dairy alternatives, such as cheese, milk and yogurt made from sheep's or goat's milk. They are lower in saturated fats on the whole, and healthier for your heart, so are a very good anti-ageing option.

Life would be very dull without cheese, so I have included those that are lower in saturated fat than the average Cheddar and tasty enough to satisfy those cheese urges. Cheese may be high in calcium but it is also very high in salt so *moderation* is the key word here. You can get calcium from far healthier sources. Using a tiny amount of cheese grated on to salads or cubed and added to a dish, you can make a huge difference to your taste buds and, if you want to continue eating animal products, it is a good source of complete protein.

## Dairy Shopping List

Butter: from cow's or goat's milk is much healthier than any of the trans fatty acids, such as margarine. It is a saturated fat, but is easily assimilated and digested because it is a 'natural' food. To be eaten in moderation.

Cottage cheese: made from skimmed milk. Not at all high in vitamins and minerals but on the approved list. Buy full fat, it is less likely to be ridden with salt and other additives.

Quark: a very low-fat cheese. It is an acquired taste, but very useful if you need a protein punch.

Vegetarian cheese: many use rennet made from cow's milk. A little of the real thing will do you more good than many of the pretend cheeses on sale.

Yogurt: calcium rich and easier to digest than milk because enzymes in its fermentation process have broken down the lactose. Make sure it is sugar-free and 'live' or 'bio' to give your gut a good dose of healthy bacteria.

Goat's cheese: ranging from hard to soft. A good buy if you suffer from lactose intolerance. Many people find an improvement in conditions such as asthma, eczema and digestive disorders when they replace cow's milk and cheese with goat's milk or cheese.

Ewe's cheese: such as halloumi is not, strictly speaking, dairy.

Buffalo mozzarella: mozzarella can be made from either cow's or buffalo milk, so for the non-dairy option make sure it's made from buffalo milk.

You don't need to be quite so anal about looking for an organic label with these cheese and yogurt alternatives because the milk comes from animals more likely to roam naturally than cows and less likely to have been fed hormones or antibiotics on a regular basis. In general these products are lower in saturated fats and healthier for your heart so are a very good anti-ageing option.

Unpasteurized cow's cheese: easier to digest and higher in nutrients, especially calcium, than pasteurized products because the heating that kills bacteria and gives cheese its long shelf life also kills many of the nutrients and healthy bacteria that raw milk contains. It shouldn't be eaten by pregnant women or anyone who has been advised by their doctor not to eat unpasteurized products.

Goat's milk: lower in fat but just as high in calcium as cow's milk and, for most people, more easily tolerated.

Rice milk: read the back of the packet as many brands contain polyunsaturated vegetable oils, which can contribute to an imbalance of the essential fats in your body. Some also contain rice syrup, cane juice or other sweeteners.

Almond milk: this is the healthiest alternative for you and your family. It is lovely and sweet, packed full of calcium (just nine almonds is the equivalent of the recommended daily allowance (RDA) of calcium needed for a fully grown man) and you can make it at home in seconds. All you need is pure water and almonds.

## NATURAL ALMOND MILK

*1½ cups raw almonds, soaked in water overnight*
*4 cups filtered or spring water*
*3–5 dates (optional)*

Whiz up the nuts and water in a blender for three minutes. Add the dates if you require more sweetness, then strain the liquid. You will have lovely, creamy milk free of artificial sweeteners, vegetable oils or dairy. It can be stored safely for three or four days in the fridge.

## Super Grains

If you are really sure wholegrain wheat does not give you a problem, then by all means add bulgar wheat, or cracked wheat, as well as wholegrain bread and pasta, to your shopping list. But, for the majority of us who do find eating wheat difficult, here are some alternatives that give you higher levels of nutrients, more proteins and less digestive problems. The best is undoubtedly any sprouted grain. After that the grains are described in order of alkalinity, with quinoa being the most alkaline and rye the most acidic.

## Super Grains Shopping List

Sprouted grains: enzymes released in the sprouting process turn into more easily digestible sugars. People who are normally intolerant to wheat are often fine with this form of wheat. High in B vitamins, potassium, magnesium, iron, zinc and phosphorus as well as selenium.

Quinoa (pronounced keen-waa): a plant of the Andes. Hailed as the mother grain because of its importance for health and longevity. Rich in calcium, magnesium and iron and contains all the essential amino acids needed to make it a complete protein all on its own. Low in starch, which keeps blood-sugar levels nice and even.

Amaranth: a herb rather than a grain. Beneficial in lowering cholesterol because of its high tocotrienol (a form of vitamin E) content. Gluten free and has three times as much fibre and five times as much iron as wheat and twice as much calcium as milk. Contains lysine and methionine, two essential amino acids that support the liver and are not normally found in grains. Cooked, it is 90 per cent digestible so is very good for recovery from illness or detoxing.

Millet: this gentle, alkaline and non-glutinous grain is high in magnesium, potassium and iron, but low in starch. It contains all eight essential amino acids.

Buckwheat: comes from a thistle plant. Its nutrient content is so similar to the other grains mentioned here that it deserves to be treated as one.

Rice: wholegrain or brown rice is packed with B vitamins and has the added bonus of containing gamma-oryzanol oil that helps heal the gut. A most efficient colon cleanser. It also gives the liver nutrients to detox.

Barley: has low levels of gluten and high levels of magnesium, calcium, iron and potassium.

Spelt: not to be confused with oats or wheat, spelt is a member of the same grain family but is an entirely different species. It does contain gluten but appears to be more easily tolerated. Bread made from spelt is very tasty, more easily digested, higher in fibre and B vitamins and 10–20 per cent higher in protein than most wheat bread.

Corn or maize: relatively high in minerals and vitamins A and C. In fact, the main source of manufactured vitamin C in America comes from fresh corn. An excellent grain for anyone who can't tolerate wheat. Polenta is made from corn and is a delicious alternative to potato or pizza.

Oats: starting the day with porridge can significantly improve your heart's health and your chances of longevity. Oats contain cancer-fighting phytoestrogens and chemicals that prevent sticky blood and lower cholesterol. Porridge also helps with blood-sugar levels as it releases energy slowly throughout the morning so you will feel fuller for longer.

Rye: contains very little gluten, which makes the bread very heavy. High in iron, potassium and magnesium. One of the most acidic grains but useful as a wheat replacement as it converts to sugar very slowly. Can be bought as pumpernickel bread.

So there are all your alternative grains. Most are higher in protein and nutrients than wheat and more easily digested and assimilated. And if you mix any one of them with pulses, you have a complete protein meal.

## Super Nuts

There are three hundred types of nuts, most of which I would consider a 'living' food because they are formed as a fruit or a seed following the flowering of a plant or tree. Nuts are one of nature's richest anti-ageing foods because they contain good quality protein, high levels of the essential fats omega-3 and 6, and vitamin E, as well as all the essential minerals such as calcium and magnesium.

Recent research findings suggest that lipase could be a key enzyme for weight loss because it helps fat to be broken down instead of being stored. Lipase is found in all high fat, 'live' foods such as nuts and seeds, especially if they are soaked first to release their enzyme activity.

Some of the nuts mentioned below are especially high in omega-3 essential fats. At the risk of repeating myself, omega-3 is needed by the body for every single cell, gland and organ. Essential fats are too essential for the body to waste them by laying them down as fat. They are used for every function of your body, including metabolism. You cannot lose weight without omega-3.

Nuts are quite hard to digest so to make them totally easy on your system, soak them for between two and twelve hours to release the enzyme inhibitors that make them more digestible. Or grind them to a fine powder before use, so they are more easily digested. Because many of the precious oils in these nuts can easily turn rancid, it is best to store them in airtight containers in the fridge or somewhere cool and dark.

## Peanuts and Cashews – No!

Peanut is not a true nut. It is more of a legume, hence the word pea in its name. Peanuts are high in protein but are also very acidic and hard to digest – and are normally salted.

Peanut butter contains hydrogenated fats, salt and sugar, so it is not a healthy spread. Instead, try almond nut butter, available in most health stores. It's far higher in anti-ageing nutrients, much lower in fat, completely natural and just as tasty.

Cashews contain low-grade oil that makes them extremely difficult to digest. A youthful, disease-free digestion needs plenty of easy-to-digest foods.

### Nut Shopping List

Walnuts: look like a brain, and that is exactly what they are good
    for because of their high omega-3 content
Hazelnuts: high in vitamin E and omega-3, therefore essential for
    healthy, young skin
Pecans: high in omega-3, antioxidants and one of the best plant
    sources of zinc for a healthy immune system
Almonds: low fat content, but extremely high in calcium; a good
    all-round nut
Brazil nuts: contain more fat than almonds but are also very high
    in selenium for a healthy thyroid and increased immunity
Pine nuts: high in protein and fibre

If your favourite nut isn't on the list, don't worry; you can
include it as long as it is not salted or a peanut or a cashew!

## Super Seeds

When it comes to anti-ageing, seeds are simply super! Plants
fill their seeds with essential fatty acids because these are the most
efficient storage form for energy – energy taken directly from the
sun. They are, quite simply, little powerhouses of nutrition providing most of the nutrients we need to keep lively, healthy and young.

### REASONS TO EAT SUPER SEEDS

- *High in essential fatty acids*
- *High levels of protein*
- *High vitamin and mineral content*
- *Can be eaten raw, cooked, ground or sprouted*
- *Keep blood-sugar levels even*

### Super Seeds Shopping List

Flaxseeds: also known as linseeds. My top seed because they are
    the richest plant source of omega-3 essential for a healthy heart,

brain, joints and skin. Known as nature's HRT because of their extremely high levels of phytoestrogens, natural plant chemicals that bind to oestrogen receptor cells in the body and mimic the hormone's effects, safely. Soaked, they are the best constipation cure I have ever come across. If you only buy one seed, make it this one.

Pumpkin seeds: high in zinc and rich in iron, calcium, phosphorus and niacin. Beneficial to men as well as women for their ability to help treat and prevent prostate problems.

Sunflower seeds: rich in potassium, as well as plenty of all the other important minerals for anti-ageing; zinc, iron and calcium. Lower in magnesium than some of the other seeds but higher in vitamin E and D. Useful for improving blood pressure, cardio-vascular problems and allergic reactions.

Hemp seeds: contain all twenty known amino acids, including the essential ones our bodies cannot produce, so are an exceptionally high-protein seed. Higher in omega-6 than 3 but in a perfect balance.

Sesame seeds: an excellent protein seed to add to grains such as rice as they are rich in some of the amino acids that grains lack. High in zinc and calcium. One tablespoon provides more than eight times the amount of calcium found in a glass of milk!

Poppy seeds: high in omega-6 while calcium and magnesium are found in abundance.

All seeds are more digestible, more alkaline and release their valu-able essential fats and nutrients better if they are soaked overnight. Otherwise, your health store or supermarket will sell big tubs of mixed seeds for you to munch on. All these seeds produce oils that will benefit your health and increase your youthfulness even more. You can find a lot more information about Super Oils in the next chapter as well as some handy tips on how they can improve your skin on page 176.

## Super Herbs and Spices

Animals instinctively search out what their bodies need when they are sick and head straight to the herbs. We also used to rely on herbs a lot more for treating illness, as well as flavouring food, than we do now. Thanks to chefs like Jamie Oliver, we're beginning to rediscover them. Herbs can be grown almost anywhere whether you have a garden or not, and are sold fresh and ready to use in most supermarkets. The first thing I did in my garden when I moved flat was to put two tubs of herbs by the door and now I take great pleasure in cutting my own to add to food all year round.

Spices are particularly important for longevity because they contain polyphenols: a group of powerful antioxidants that have for centuries been used to stop food oxidizing or going off. These nutrients are found in rosemary (rosmaric acid) and turmeric (curcumin). There has been so much research carried out on curcumin, I have to give turmeric its own space.

### Turmeric – The Top Anti-Ageing Spice

Turmeric is a member of the ginger family and with its rich anti-inflammatory, antioxidant properties is linked to the good health of the elderly in parts of the world where they are less prone to neurodegenerative diseases. In research, turmeric has been found to:

> Prevent free radical formation
> Neutralize existing free radicals
> Possibly reduce the risk of Alzheimer's
> Lower cholesterol
> Protect the liver

Which all adds up to a perfect prescription for healthy and youthful ageing and a great excuse to order an Indian curry, if you don't have time to make it from scratch!

## Salt

Despite my earlier comments about salt there are a couple of salts that have been recommended to me by naturopathic doctors that bear no relation to the stuff from the supermarket. Sodium is essential for the electrolyte balance of the cells and when you consider that a sperm cell consists of 99 per cent water and 1 per cent sodium, that's a good enough reason to use a little of the right type.

### 'Good' Salts

Nature et Progrès Seasalt is harvested by hand with no added chemicals and none of its minerals or electrolytes removed. It is low in organic sodium and has the right ratios of magnesium, potassium and calcium for an alkaline balance. As it's unrefined, it is grey in colour and slightly damp. Dr Shamim Daya, who specializes in nutritional medicine, says this salt is the one exception to the rule because, 'It is as nature intended and includes essential minerals such as potassium, which will help balance your body.'

Another recommended salt is a pink, crystal salt from the Himalayas that contains all eight essential minerals. As it is crystalline, all the elements that benefit your health are trapped within the salt and are in such small particles they are able to penetrate the cells and be metabolized. This is the salt I use. It has such a strong flavour I only need a tiny amount.

Both these salts can be found in the better health stores or on-line (see Resources, page 235 for Himalayan crystal salt). There are other equally harmless salts. The best advice I can give is to look for one that is unrefined, not white but grey or pink in colour and slightly damp in texture.

## Super Herbs and Spices Shopping List

Cayenne: natural anti-inflammatory
Ginger: natural anti-inflammatory, warms the body, aids digestion, helps stop travel sickness and helps the liver detox

Caraway seeds: good for indigestion and menstrual cramps

Chilli: helps detox and is a decongestant, rich in vitamin C

Black pepper: stimulates digestive juices

Cinnamon: relieves stomach upsets, cold and flu symptoms and 1 teaspoon daily has been found to lower cholesterol levels as efficiently as statins do

Nettles: incredibly high in calcium, magnesium, manganese, and iron. Pick young shoots and boil to make tea or soup

Milk thistle: liver cleansing and detoxing

Comfrey: use externally for rheumatism, painful joints, muscles, ligaments

Aloe vera: the juice from the leaves can be used to relieve sunburn and skin complaints – use it internally for a healthy digestion

Coriander: good for cramp and flatulence

Fennel: a natural anti-bloater, contains oestragole, an oestrogen-like compound

Cumin: good for stopping diarrhoea

Garlic: a powerful detoxifier

Onion: helps the liver detox

## Super Sea Vegetables

Sea vegetables are the foods richest in the minerals we need for anti-ageing and prime health. Gillian McKeith, author of *Living Food for Health*, says they contain twelve key minerals not found anywhere else in plant form, including magnesium, sodium, calcium and potassium. They also contain high concentrations of iodine, which maintains thyroid health, chlorine and manganese, good for the pituitary gland, zinc which benefits the immune system and iron for healthy blood.

According to Gillian McKeith, the protein in seaweed is more easily absorbed by the body than the protein found in meat or fish, making it one of nature's best anti-ageing foods on the planet. It is alkaline, so will make our bodies less acidic, and a more alkaline body is a younger body.

Seaweed is a form of marine algae that grows in the upper levels of the sea producing 70 per cent of the earth's oxygen. There are literally hundreds of species but only a dozen or so that we can actually eat. Here are a few of the more common ones you should be able to buy in health stores:

## Sea Vegetables Shopping List

Arame: rich in magnesium, potassium, calcium, sodium and iodine
Kelp: one teaspoon has a *thousand* times more calcium than a glass of milk as well as being iodine rich.
Wakami: rich in iron and ten times more calcium than a glass of milk.
Nori: twice as much vitamin C as oranges, as much beta-carotene as carrots, and rich in B vitamins, calcium for your bones, iron and iodine for your thyroid. You can buy nori flakes or get sheets of nori to make sushi.
Dulse: contains fifteen times more calcium than cow's milk and eight times the amount of iron found in beef.

Sea vegetables are available from good health shops or on-line. They come dried and ready to use. If you feel really adventurous you could go to a beach or a fishmonger to find fresh seaweed and try cooking this:

### SEAWEED JELLY CAKES

Scottish seaweed connoisseurs recommend washing fresh seaweed and soaking it for two hours. Simmer in a covered saucepan for three to four hours until it becomes a jelly. Drain, beat well with butter and add one to two tablespoons each of lemon and orange juice. Season with salt and pepper, mix in a little oatmeal until stiff, shape into flat cakes and fry.

Hopefully, you now have a long list of anti-ageing foods to add to your usual weekly shop. One of the most important groups of nutrients are the essential fats found in oily fish, nuts and seeds. Unfortunately, not everyone can eat them. An extremely potent and easy way of adding more EFAs to your diet, especially if you are a vegetarian or vegan, is to use oils made from the nuts and seeds rich in omega-3 and 6.

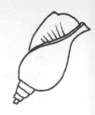

4.

# Super Fats, Super Oils

## *Essential Fatty Acids (EFAs) Omega-3 and Omega-6*

Because we have come to associate fats with ill health and piling on the pounds, clients usually have a fit when I start cajoling them to include more essential fats in their diets. So let's get rid of that misapprehension straightaway! You *cannot* lose weight effectively without omega-3 and 6 because of their effect on the metabolism. EFAs increase your energy levels, decrease your stress levels and improve your skin's appearance. Once you start eating them regularly you will never be without them again.

All fats, or lipids, are needed by the body to produce energy and to protect and insulate our vital organs. I'm not talking about saturated fats such as those found in cheese, lard, suet, bacon and fatty meats. We all know they go straight onto our thighs and cause heart disease if eaten in excess. Hydrogenated fats such as margarines can also affect our long-term health even more than saturated fat because they are trans fatty acids, which produce free radicals.

Essential fats, on the other hand, make up the membranes of every single cell in the body and dictate the state of your health and appearance. They control how well your cells cope with what is flowing in and out of them: oxygen, fluid, nutrients and toxins. Within each cell are receptor sites where vital hormones such as insulin and neurotransmitters such as serotonin communicate. If those cell membranes are too rigid because of a lack of EFAs the chemicals cannot dock and deliver their messages. This results in, for example, blood-sugar problems from insulin imbalance or depression because of a serotonin deficiency.

The three essential fatty acids our bodies need to convert into something it can use are: arachidonic, alpha-linolenic (omega-3) and linoleic (omega-6) acids. We can't make them ourselves and have to rely on our food to provide them. Because of our modern eating habits, most of us have an abundance of arachidonic acid, found in meat, dairy and eggs, enough omega-6 from grains, fruit and vegetables, but nowhere near enough omega-3 needed in highly concentrated amounts for our brain cells, eyes, adrenal glands and nerves. We consumed enough omega-3 when we were hunter-gatherers but, because our consumption of oily fish has declined by a staggering 80 per cent in the last hundred years, we are way out of balance and showing signs of an omega-3 deficiency.

## OMEGA-3 DEFICIENCY SYMPTOMS

- *Depression*
- *Hormonal problems*
- *Dry skin*
- *Flaking nails*
- *Dull hair*
- *Tiredness*
- *Vaginal dryness*
- *Painful intercourse*
- *Premature ageing*
- *Arthritis*
- *Water retention*
- *Seasonal affective disorder*
- *Blood-sugar blues*

An oil high in omega-3 and 6 essential fatty acids will help relieve all of the above symptoms so you age healthily and look youthful. It can make the difference between a soft complexion and one like a bit of old leather!

## Benefits of Omega-3 and 6

Skin and hair health: EFAs are a natural moisturizer. Omega-3-rich oils improve the skin's condition and help it stay young, healthy and flexible.

Metabolism: EFAs speed up the metabolism and transfer oxygen to the cells more effectively, helping you burn fuel more efficiently so you lose weight.

Heart health: omega-3 has been shown in many studies to lower triglycerides and cholesterol levels, decrease blood pressure and prevent hardening of the arteries.

Hormonal balance: flaxseeds (and therefore flaxseed oil) are particularly high in phytoestrogens which mimic natural oestrogen in your body, safely.

Healthy bowels: consuming more omega-3 has proved a major success for patients suffering from all manner of bowel problems, from diverticulosis to constipation.

Seasonal affective disorder (SAD): helps absorb sunlight.

The sun's rays reach the earth as a source of energy on which all the earth's minerals, plants and foods rely. The photon is the tiniest part of a sunbeam and is recognized as being the purest form of energy. Electrons love photons and are attracted to them like moths to a light. Oils made from seeds are packed full of these electrons and will help you absorb some of that sun's light and energy. This is why these oils are particularly important for any of us living in the northern latitudes with our long dark winters and lack of light.

Most of the seed and nut oils mentioned in this section are a potent source of omega-3 and are a healthy alternative for those who can't eat oily fish regularly, but there is one warning. Omega-3 has to be converted in the body from alpha-linolenic acid to EPA and DHA, the two essential fatty acids found in oily fish. The body uses an enzyme called delta-6 to make this conversion, but it is found in lower levels in women, older people, or people under stress, so you may want to take two EPA fish oil capsules a day, as well as using one of the oils, to reap maximum benefits. Unless, of course, you are a vegetarian or vegan.

Apart from the omega-3 and 6 oils, there are other interesting nut oils and cooking oils in this chapter, some of which are exotic and unusual. They are all, however, packed full of nutrients and will improve the health of every cell in your body if used regularly.

## Seed Oils

All the oils mentioned in this section should be kept in dark, cool places because they oxidize easily. Many of them cannot be used for cooking because heating makes them unstable. You will probably have to get these oils from a health-food shop, delicatessen or through mail order, unless your supermarket is very well stocked.

One to two tablespoons a day will give your body all it needs in the way of omega-3 and 6 essential fats. You can add them to smoothies, drizzle them onto hot food, use them in salad dressing or dunk some wheat-free bread into them.

### Flaxseed Oil

The richest source of omega-3 is found in flaxseeds and flaxseed oil so it is at the top of the Super Oils list. It also contains small amounts of the other essential fatty acid we can't make ourselves: omega-6. You may find flaxseed oil an acquired taste, or you may love it. It *cannot* be heated. I have managed to find a completely tasteless one (see Resources, page 234), which I use for salad dressings along with a teaspoon or two of olive oil.

Flaxseed oil will benefit the health of every cell in your body and give you a lovely soft skin, especially if you use it topically, as recommended in the Super Skin chapter.

Make sure you buy good-quality flaxseed oil that is cold-pressed and sold in a lightproof bottle.

### Hempseed Oil

Dr Udo Erasmus, the world's leading expert on oils and author of the book *Fats That Heal, Fats That Kill*, considers hempseed oil to be nature's most perfectly balanced oil due to its high content of both omega-3 and omega-6. Despite its origins, it is completely legal and safe!

It contains more omega-6 fats but is as effective as flaxseed oil for maintaining heart health and reducing a cholesterol build-up. Hempseed oil is particularly good for skin complaints such as eczema and I have used it with great success in my clinic for treating many skin conditions. Hempseeds are also the only seeds to contain GLA, an essential fatty acid that is ideal for treating PMS. I particularly recommend using this oil during the summer months because we don't need as much omega-3 at that time of the year as we get plenty of light from the longer daylight hours.

Hempseed oil is cold-pressed and has a sweet, nutty flavour, nicer than the taste of flaxseed oil. It should *not* be heated but can be used as a salad dressing, as a butter substitute, drizzled onto your food, or put in a smoothie.

### Pumpkinseed Oil

Pumpkinseed oil is rich in omega-3 and 6, vitamins E and A which are good for the skin and zinc for boosting the immune system. It may alleviate bladder and prostate problems. It is considered one of the top three oils providing the highest EFAs for a healthy young mind and body. It is less widely available than the previous two oils.

This oil also *cannot* be heated and is best added to a smoothie or used as a salad dressing. It is tasty oil and keeps better than flaxseed oil and rarely goes rancid. This one is worth a try if you like more exotic oils.

### Sesame Oil

Sesame oil is highly flavoured and contains high amounts of vitamins E and B, as well as all the important anti-ageing minerals and essential fats. It is also high in lecithin, for healthy brain cells, nerves and energy. The oil that is pressed from these tiny seeds is rich and golden in colour with a delicious nutty taste.

The dark version of this oil should not be used for cooking because it burns easily. But the lighter oil, made from unroasted sesame seeds, *can be* used for stir-frying and is often used in Indian cookery.

### Grapeseed Oil

Grapeseed oil is one of the most stable cooking oils and, as a by-product of wine production, has been popular with European chefs for hundreds of years. It is well known for its high antioxidant content which protects against heart disease and helps clear fatty deposits from the blood. It is one of the few natural foods known to raise 'healthy' HDL cholesterol levels. It is also high in omega-6 as well as containing decent amounts of vitamin E and bioflavonoids that will help protect you against free radicals.

This oil can be heated to high temperatures without affecting its flavour and without burning or smoking. It is one of the most stable of cooking oils and doesn't splatter like so many others. It has such a subtle flavour it can be used for deep or shallow frying (if you must!) and is ideal for strongly flavoured foods such as fish. You need less of it than other cooking oils, so it is more economical.

## Nut Oils

Nut oils, like the nuts they are pressed from, are very low in saturated fats and bursting with anti-ageing benefits. Almond, hazel, macadamia and pecan nut oils are high in monounsaturated fats, which help lower 'bad' cholesterol; walnut oil is rich in polyunsaturates and omega-3 essential fats for protecting your heart; and

argan, almond and hazelnut oils are rich in vitamin E for beautiful skin.
**If you suffer from a nut allergy do not use any of these oils.**

## Argan Oil

Argan oil is one of my very favourite 'speciality' oils to make a starter or a salad that little bit different. It is extracted from the Moroccan argan tree and has been used by the Berber women for centuries to serve for breakfast, with freshly baked bread, sprinkled on salads and vegetables or tagines and couscous. It has a delicious, rich, nutty flavour and is being heralded by chefs like Antony Worrall Thompson as the new 'trendy' oil.

Health-wise argan oil is superb. Like all other nut oils, it is very low in saturated fats, as well as having a good profile of omega-6 essential fats. Argan oil contains almost twice as much vitamin E as olive oil, is rich in antioxidants and contains rare plant sterols, not found in other oils, that give it anti-inflammatory properties that have successfully helped treat rheumatic joint pain, blocked arteries and high cholesterol. It is also good for liver and gall bladder health.

Externally, argan oil is used by Moroccan women for protecting and nourishing their skin and has been used successfully to reduce scarring, acne and psoriasis. The vitamin E content is so high that you will find this oil in the Super Skin section as a recommended moisturizer (see page 176).

This is another oil that must *not* be heated, but it is so delicious that I urge you to try it if you get the chance. It is much better combined with lemon or lime juice, rather than vinegar, and is fantastic in a rocket and goat's cheese or grated Parmesan salad. However, as it takes 30 kg of nuts and ten hours' work to produce just one litre of oil, it is more of an expensive 'treat' than an everyday oil. I mix mine with olive oil to make it go further.

But please, only buy argan oil from the website mentioned in Resources on page 234 as the producers are working alongside the Berbers to ensure their traditional way of life is not destroyed.

## Walnut Oil

Nut oils such as walnut and hazelnut add a distinct flavour to bread, salads and cooking. The most commonly used in the UK is walnut oil and, apart from being extremely high in omega-3, it contains an antioxidant compound called ellagic acid which has been found to inhibit the growth of cancer cells.

The oil has the flavour of crushed walnuts and works very well in salad dressing, especially with more unusual vinegars such as sherry. If you use it in baking you get the taste of the nuts. Walnut oil is *not* suitable for frying.

## Other Nut Oils

The following nut oils are not as easy to come by in the UK and are quite pricey, but they are worth a try if you want to add the flavour of the nuts to your food.

Almond: recommended for sautéing and stir-frying, although it seems more popular as a skin-care oil! High in calcium.

Hazelnut: like walnut oil, hazelnut oil tastes of the nuts it comes from and is rich and tasty. It is quite strong so you only need a little to add a bit of oomph to a salad dressing. It can also be used for baking. High in omega-3.

Macadamia: a delicate oil that goes well with fish or vegetables. Drizzle some on before serving.

Pecan: like walnut and hazelnut oils, pecan oil tastes of nuts and is high in omega-3. Try it in dressings, drizzled on vegetables or in baking.

# Cooking Oils

## Olive Oil

Olive oil is the most commonly used 'healthy' oil for cooking, particularly if it is extra virgin olive oil. Olives and olive oil have been around for thousands of years. Hippocrates prescribed olive oil for curing ulcers, gallbladder problems, muscle aches and many other conditions. More recently, olive oil was the first oil to be associated with 'good' fats. Its high monounsaturated fat content has been publicized widely for its ability to cut cholesterol and combat heart disease.

The first cold-pressed (extra virgin) olive oil is the best grade with less acidity and the highest levels of fatty acids and poly-phenols – powerful antioxidants found in the soil where olives are grown – especially around the Mediterranean. One of the reasons for its high antioxidant content is that the olive is exposed to the air and produces a larger number of antioxidants to protect itself and these get passed on to the oil you use.

Olive oil is an important part of a wrinkle-free programme because of its vitamin E and polyphenol content, making it a very potent anti-inflammatory food and one that appears to contribute to longevity in the countries where it is consumed daily.

It is more fattening than the omega-3-rich oils so I only use a little in relation to flaxseed oil, for example, 1 teaspoon of olive oil to 1 tablespoon of flaxseed oil for salad dressings. For cooking, a little goes a long way.

## Avocado Oil

Avocado oil is a smooth, rich, extra virgin oil extracted from my favourite fruit. As an oil, it is a relative newcomer, but one that is becoming more popular. It tastes nutty and is rich in vitamin E for healthy skin, vitamin D for healthy bones and vitamin A for healthy eyes, hair and nails.

Studies have shown that avocado oil can reduce the risk of type 2 diabetes and prostate problems. It can be used cold or for searing food at high temperatures as it has a high smoke point. It can be drizzled over meat, fish or vegetables before roasting or to make salad dressings, marinades or to use instead of butter.

Try adding lemon, rosemary or chilli and use it to add flavour to mashed potato (preferably sweet potato!) or for drizzling over steamed vegetables. Yum!

## Coconut Oil

Finally, a saturated fat that is considered so beneficial it has to go under Super Fats. Coconut oil has, for many decades, received some very bad press because of its saturated-fat content. A major study was conducted over forty years ago, using hydrogenated oil not *virgin* coconut oil – the only one I would recommend.

More recent research has shown that coconut oil is not like the other 'bad' fats because it also contains the highest source of saturated *medium* chain triglycerides of any naturally occurring vegan food source, half of which are made up of lauric acid that some anti-ageing experts consider the most important essential fatty acid for building and maintaining a strong immune system. Medium chain fatty acids do not elevate cholesterol in the way that other saturated fats can.

The only other source of lauric acid, apart from small amounts in milk fat and butter, is in mother's milk. Rather than doing the body harm, lauric acid has powerful antiviral and antibacterial properties, and is converted to the anti-ageing steroids, pregnenolone, progesterone and DHEA: the youth hormones that prevent heart disease, senility, obesity and chronic degeneration.

The medium chain fatty acids found in virgin coconut oil also help to increase metabolism by supporting the thyroid and are more easily digested than other saturated fats because they are immediately converted to energy. This is such a healthy, non-fattening, youth-promoting oil that I now use it for cooking more than olive oil, especially for baking. But it must be unrefined and virgin. Coconut oil comes in a solid form when you buy it, so leave it out in a warm kitchen if you are going to use it for baking and refrigerate once it's opened.

Coconut butter is also worth buying as it is considered an excellent dietary fat for people with Candida, hormone imbalances and low blood-sugar levels. It contains powerful anti-viral and anti-fungal properties but no cholesterol, trans fatty acids or hydrogenated fats. It is a perfect alternative to butter for vegans and vegetarians.

*

That completes a brief look at all the nutrient-rich and anti-ageing oils that can be used for cooking, drizzling over food or for using in a salad dressing. The next chapter, Super Drinks, will show you how to add them to smoothies so you can make a meal on the run that will give your body everything it needs in one glass.

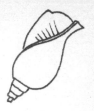

# 5.
# Super Drinks

Drinks are far more than just drinks when it comes to anti-ageing. In the words of Mahatma Gandhi, if you want a healthy digestion and body, 'eat your drinks and drink your food!' The more liquid the food in the form of smoothies, juices and soups, the less energy the body needs to digest them. The less energy the body needs to use, the more energy is available for it to cleanse and renew itself and the healthier your cells will be. The healthier your cells are, the younger you look and feel!

## Super Smoothies

You will have seen why vegetable oils are so important in anti-ageing but it makes them even more effective when added to a smoothie that will make a filling, nutrient-rich meal replacement. All you need is a blender and your preferred fruits. You can have a smoothie for breakfast, lunch or supper; perfect for anyone who hasn't the time or the energy to prepare a meal.

### Fruit Juice

Any fruit juice can be used for your smoothie, as long as it doesn't contain added sugar. Although not as high in nutrients as fresh fruit there are many juices on sale that are packed with nothing other than fresh fruit: apple, mango, cranberry to name but three. If you are really short of time, you can buy a ready-made smoothie and keep it in the fridge. Some of the best ones are readily available and contain pure, low-sugar, high-antioxidant berries such as blueberries and strawberries. Look for one that is made from 100 per cent pure unadulterated fruit, without additives, preservatives, colourings or sugar.

## Fruit

Berries are best! Berries are the top anti-ageing fruit, high in antioxidants and water, but low in sugar. They are also easy to buy frozen, so you can eat them out of season. And of course you can always pick your own, in season, and freeze them yourself. You only need a handful for each smoothie and, if you add another magic ingredient, lecithin (see page 91), they have the capacity to turn an ordinary smoothie into a really creamy milkshake without any milk.

## Omega-3 and 6 Oil

Choose flaxseed, hempseed or an omega-3/6 blended oil, available from health stores and some supermarkets, to put in a smoothie and be prepared for a boost in energy and a completely suppressed appetite. This is the one ingredient that will take energy straight into your cells, especially if you add one of the recommended proteins (see below) to the drink. The EFAs in the oils help your kidneys dump excess water and suppress your appetite as well as making your blood-sugar levels more stable, putting an end to cravings. You will feel full for longer than you expect with two tablespoons of oil in your smoothie. And don't forget, they do *not* make you put on weight, they do quite the reverse and help speed up your metabolism. And they make your skin looked plumped-up and young.

## Protein

A tablespoon of quark, cottage cheese or ground nuts or seeds is also recommended as an additional ingredient to a smoothie for several reasons. Protein is very important for supporting the liver and adrenal glands so your body will function better, especially in the morning. A small portion of protein will also make the smoothie more substantial and keep you feeling full for longer.

But the most important reason for including this particular type of protein is because of the way it interacts with whatever seed oil you choose, to give you more energy. Dr Johanna Budwig, seven times Nobel prize nominee and considered to be one of the foremost authorities on fats and healing, recommends that essential fats should be put together with cottage cheese or quark because they help the oils dissolve more easily. When you mix one of the recommended oils with one of these proteins, the amino acid cysteine, present in quark, cottage cheese and nuts and seeds, makes the fat become water-soluble. This makes it rich in electrons, which carry more energy, light and oxygen into your cells. Dr Budwig likens it to recharging a dead battery. So give your smoothie a protein punch and an anti-ageing blast.

## Lecithin Granules

Lecithin is a nutrient and oil found in most living tissues, especially the liver and brain. It forms part of the cell membrane as a phospholipid and plays an essential part in making your cells strong, flexible and healthy, allowing nutrients to flow in and toxins to flow out.

Lecithin is very rich in omega-6. Because of its high choline content, lecithin also protects your brain, helps you retain your memory and is renowned for getting rid of hangovers! It protects and helps regenerate the liver and, most important of all, lecithin is a fat emulsifier so helps reduce cholesterol in your body as well as acting like washing-up liquid in your smoothie. Lecithin granules break down the fat in the oil so the whole thing turns into a creamy, milkshake-like drink without a trace of oil.

Start with one to three heaped teaspoons of lecithin and build up to a dessertspoon if you like it and feel good on it. Some people need time for their livers to adjust to lecithin, while others just love it. Listen to your body and if you feel at all sick, reduce the amount.

Lecithin granules can be found in any reputable health store. They can be extracted from eggs, soybeans or corn, so check the source and make sure it is not genetically modified.

## SUPER SMOOTHIE

*1–2 tablespoons flaxseed, hempseed or an omega-3/6 blended oil*
*a glass of fruit juice (not orange as it can be too acidic)*
*a handful of mixed berries: blueberries, strawberries and raspberries*
*1 teaspoon to 1 dessertspoon lecithin granules*
*1 tablespoon quark, cottage cheese or ground seeds and nuts*
*½ a banana, if needed*

Put all the ingredients in the blender, whizz and drink. If it isn't sweet enough, you might like to add a couple of dates or a spoonful of honey. It should keep you going for hours.

## Super Water

It's not the cells that cause ageing; it's the liquid in the cells. We're made up of 75 per cent water, slopping around in our blood, tissues, organs and bones. All of it is absolutely vital in order for the body to carry out its many functions and keep us looking youthful and thinking clearly. Water carries nutrients and oxygen into our cells, and removes the body's waste. It also transports sodium, calcium, magnesium, potassium and other salts in and out of the cell membranes for the electrolyte balance, without which nothing functions as well as it should. Next to the air we breathe, water is the most important substance we will ever put in our bodies.

Water helps dilute acids, making the blood more alkaline and the internal system healthier. It moisturizes the skin, surrounds every joint and bone in the body, and is essential for brain health. The brain has more than fifteen billion cells that need water and oxygen to function at maximum capacity. We sometimes forget that the brain is an organ – an organ almost entirely made up of water and essential fats.

The body becomes chronically and increasingly dehydrated the older we get. A dry mouth is the very last sign of dehydration. According to Mu Shik Jhon, PhD, a world authority on water,

'Hydration is directly related to your health, skin and ageing.' There is no doubt that the ageing process can be improved by increasing the body's hydration and alkalinity.

While all doctors agree that water is very important, it is now becoming more widely known that water can actually be used to treat and improve certain conditions such as diabetes, arthritis, obesity, headaches, hypertension and heart disease. Every single vertebra is surrounded by water, so if you want a healthy, pain-free back in old age, start drinking more water now!

Finally, the colon is where the body has a huge percentage of its water to bulk up waste and help move it along and out of the body. The more water you drink the more often you will move your bowels and the less waste and toxicity will be left in the body to fester and age you.

## BENEFITS OF DRINKING WATER

- *Balances electrolytes*
- *Encourages bowel movement*
- *Moves toxins out of the body more quickly*
- *Makes blood more alkaline*
- *Helps kidneys excrete acids*
- *Makes skin look younger*
- *Relieves stress*
- *Lubricates bones and joints*
- *Reduces cholesterol*
- *Helps blood pressure*
- *Prevents headaches*
- *Helps digestive juices work*
- *Maintains blood-sugar levels*
- *Prevents hangovers*
- *Prevents fatigue*
- *Helps prevent allergic reactions*

## Won't Other Fluids Do?

In a word – no! What is the first thing you check if you have a dog, cat or any other pet? The water bowl. If you have a garden or just a few plants around your home, what do you give them? Water! Some dogs enjoy a bowl of beer – occasionally. Some gardeners swear by putting tea leaves on their plants – occasionally. And some cats love cream – occasionally. But, as their main fluid, they all need water and so do we.

Coffee, tea, wine and beer don't count because we actually need to increase our intake of water to make up for the dehydration they cause (apart from some herbal teas). Rehydration expert, Dr Susan Shirreffs, explains, 'Tea, coffee, cola or anything that contains caffeine may act as a diuretic and stimulate urination. Alcohol has an even stronger diuretic effect than caffeine.' Every time you drink a cup of coffee, tea or alcohol, you are encouraging your kidneys to take more fluid out of your body than you put in.

## How Much Should I Drink?

We lose nearly 2 litres of water from our bodies every day without doing anything. Fluid is lost through perspiration, breathing, coughing, pooing and weeing. Just being. So we need to replace that amount of lost water as a bare minimum. We need to replace even more if we are exercising or leading a very stressful life.

As a matter of course, I would recommend at least 1.5–3 litres of fluid a day (including juices and herbal teas). Two litres is a happy medium and is only eight glasses of water a day – that's one an hour. You will know if you are drinking enough by having a quick look at your urine. Apart from first thing, when the body will be dehydrated, you should be aiming for straw-coloured urine – a very pale yellow.

If you are new to drinking more water, make sure you pick a time to increase your intake when you are at home and near a loo rather than a busy period when you are out and about all the time. The bladder adapts to an increase in water more quickly than you imagine. It may take a week or two, but as your body becomes more and more hydrated it will *want* more and more water and you may find, for the first time in your life, that you actually develop a taste and a thirst for it.

I used to find drinking plain water boring, but my body soon changed and I was surprised to find that I soon 'craved' my glasses of water. The only thing that makes me rush to the loo now is coffee or alcohol!

## ADVICE FOR DRINKING MORE WATER

- *Drink still water. Fizzy water is bloating and over-filling.*
- *Drink it at room temperature, it's easier to get down.*
- *Don't drink water with your meals – it interferes with the digestion.*
- *Drink water no later than 30 minutes before a meal.*
- *Don't drink for 1–2 hours after a meal.*
- *Don't drink more than ½ litre of water at once as it can overload the kidneys.*
- *Don't drink more than 2 litres in an hour, for the same reason.*
- *Don't drink after 9 p.m. if you want an undisturbed night.*

## Types of Water

### Tap Water
This usually tastes disgusting and carries up to 300 different kinds of pesticide and fungicide residues! The ever-present fluoride has also been blamed, by thyroid specialists, for suppressing this important gland's function and possibly contributing to the epidemic of under-functioning thyroids.

### Natural Mineral and Spring Water
By law this water has to come from a natural source at which it is bottled, and it must have a constant composition. It is not processed so it is, by definition, natural. But check the labels very carefully and make sure it is low in calcium and sodium and higher in magnesium and potassium. Natural spring water is usually

stored in plastic bottles so to save both your pocket and the environment, consider one of the other systems described below.

### Jug Water Filter

The cheapest and easiest home-filter option which uses activated carbon to filter chemicals out of the tap water. Filters are much more affordable than they used to be, but they only filter a limited amount of water at a time and the filter needs changing regularly. However, it is cheaper and more environmentally friendly than buying all those plastic bottles.

### Under the Sink Filter

This is much more expensive but worth considering if you value your health. Once the system is installed, the price of 2 litres of water a day works out much cheaper than buying bottles. It is worth looking around for one of the many filters produced in Japan. Researchers there have carried out some of the most detailed studies into water in the world and have helped design filters that imitate natural aerated water flowing down a mountain, by filtering it through alkaline minerals. As well as filtering out most of the chemicals in tap water, a good, under the sink filter will oxygenate your water and increase its alkalinity.

### Reverse Osmosis

This is even more expensive but excludes almost 100 per cent of the impurities found in water, including fluoride. However, it also re-moves virtually all the naturally occurring minerals, which we need.

### Distilled Water

Expensive and the unit takes up space. The jury is out on this one. Some experts say this is the very purest water on the planet because it contains none of the inorganic minerals found in tap and mineral water and none of the poisons and pollutants found in tap water. Others say it is too pure and could 'leach' precious minerals out of our bodies just as pure rainwater leaches minerals from the rocks.

*

So those are the main types of water you can drink. As long as you get water down you I don't think you need to lose sleep over what type of water you are drinking – as long as it's water. Just choose the method and type that is most convenient for you and your purse. I have finally bought an under the sink filter and am thrilled to pieces that I can now drink good, oxygenated water, use it for making hot drinks and cook with it.

## Super Juices

Juicing fresh vegetables is just the very best thing you can do if you want younger cells. When you juice, you are extracting 90 per cent of those anti-ageing nutrients and taking them straight into every cell in your body. That compares to obtaining only 50 per cent of the nutrients if you eat raw vegetables and even less if you cook them.

Remember that plants convert the sun's energy to produce chlorophyll. When we drink our greens we are therefore taking in some of the sun's energy that will, in turn, give us high octane fuel energy. Vegetables are, as you have already seen, mostly alkaline and an alkaline body is a young body.

So, if you have a juicer, here are a few suggestions you may not have considered. If you don't have a juicer, don't worry, just eat more raw veg and skip this section. However, the price of juicers is coming down, so it may be worth you putting one on your Christmas list.

When it comes to buying vegetables to juice, it is important that you buy organic wherever possible as you will be getting 90 per cent of any chemicals they may contain. Always wash, top and tail the veg, and peel anything not organic.

The first juice recommended is a liver flush. There is plenty more on why looking after your liver helps you age better in the Super Bod chapter but suffice to say that regularly drinking juice helps your liver detox, which will help you look younger as well as feeling more energized. Hot flushes, skin eruptions and a dull, lacklustre appearance are just some of the many signs that the liver is under stress and needs a little kick-start.

The best foods for helping the liver detox are beetroot, radishes, watercress and ginger, because they help drain the liver by stimulating the gall bladder. If you are feeling very brave, add 1 dessertspoon of olive oil and freshly squeezed lemon juice to this mixture. The phytonutrients in the olive oil will help the liver produce antioxidants and the lemon juice will kick-start this important anti-ageing organ. A liver flush can be carried out when you are detoxing, for example straight after Christmas, or when you are following one of the anti-ageing diets. Just remember that any form of juicing will get your cells to unload like mad so may cause detox symptoms such as headaches, fatigue and spots, so do take care. Just listen to your body and stop if you feel at all unwell.

If you are reading this and *don't* have a juicer, freshly squeezed lemon juice in hot water is also a fantastic liver help and will do the job nearly as well, without major detoxing. It will also make your system nice and alkaline.


## LIVER FLUSH

*1 small beetroot*
*4 carrots*
*4 sticks celery*
*handful of fresh watercress*
*6 radishes*
*chunk of ginger*
*1–2 apples to sweeten*
*1 dessertspoon extra virgin olive oil (optional)*
*2 teaspoons freshly squeezed lemon juice (optional)*

There are plenty of other vegetables to use for juicing, so experiment and see how you get on. The only *fruits* recommended for juicing are lemons, oranges and apples. Fruits, such as berries, aren't really suitable as so much of the goodness in the skin is just wasted. Strawberries make very little juice, so save your money and pop them into smoothies instead.

## Suggested Juicing Veg

Carrot: Czech researchers have found that carrots contain a substance similar to caffeine without the disadvantages!

Red cabbage: sweet and high in glutamine, which helps restore the digestive tract.

All greens: a little bitter, but high in all four essential minerals, calcium, magnesium, potassium and sodium. Makes the system alkaline.

Lemon: juice some of the rind along with the flesh as it is rich in bioflavonoids as well as vitamin C.

Beetroot: high in natural chlorine which cleanses liver, kidneys and gall bladder.

Cucumber: a natural diuretic and rich in silicon and sulphur for strong skin, nails and hair.

Celery: a diuretic also high in organic sodium to help toxin elimination.

Parsley: a diuretic and adrenal gland supporter, high in calcium and vitamin C.

Fennel: a liver and digestion stimulant that shifts toxins and clears the skin.

Radishes: high in glyconutrients for boosting immunity.

Red, yellow or orange peppers: high in beta-carotene for free-radical protection.

## Wheatgrass

This is the lazy person's version of a vegetable juice. I am using wheatgrass at the moment because it is so quick to prepare and packs a nutritional punch like no other vegetable. One shot is equivalent to 1½ kilos of vegetables, in nutrients. This is the easiest way to obtain a huge burst of anti-agers in one tiny shot.

The downside is that you need to find somewhere selling trays of this wonder grass (it is very easy to grow your own) and it has a very strong taste that can make many people feel extremely sick – usually those who are very toxic. So this is *not* the juice to drink if you feel your liver is overloaded, as it will just pay you back with a double dose of biliousness.

If you have a juicer you will need to check whether you can use it to juice wheatgrass, as not all of them are suitable. There are, however, special little juicer-like contraptions on sale in health shops especially for wheatgrass. They are very reasonably priced but don't juice any other vegetables, being manual not electrical. If all else fails, there are juice bars up and down the country so you can pop in and have a quick fix of wheatgrass there.

The use of wheatgrass goes back to the Old Testament. When a king lost his physical and mental health, he heard a voice telling him to eat the grass as an ox eats. The king followed this advice and regained his health. Instead of *eating* grass, get a tray of this beautiful, lush greenery, juice a handful of wheatgrass and try it daily for a couple of weeks. I add an orange or two to mine to hide the taste and find it as energizing as a quick jog up and down the beach! It is a 'living' food, so feeds oxygen directly into the body to help you feel strong, healthy and happy.

## WHEAT GRASS BENEFITS

- *High in vitamins A, D and B*
- *High in calcium, phosphorus, iron, potassium, sulphur, sodium, cobalt and zinc*
- *Contains all essential amino acids*
- *A complete protein equal to eating twenty-five hamburgers*
- *Chlorophyll increases the function of heart, intestines and lungs*
- *High in phycomin – natural happy chemicals*
- *High in oxygen – needed for the brain, body tissues and energy*
- *High in magnesium – an essential anti-ageing mineral*
- *Improves blood-sugar fluctuations*
- *Can stop the hair from greying*
- *Helps bowel movements*
- *Reduces high blood pressure*

- *Strengthens capillaries – essential for a young skin*
- *Helps remove heavy metals from the body*

## Super Hot Drinks

### Coffee

Enough has been said about the dos and don'ts of drinking coffee in the Super Agers chapter. It is a drink that many of us cannot get through the day without, and I completely understand if you are not prepared to live without your one cup a day. If you are trying to substitute coffee with something healthier and wheatgrass or juiced carrots don't work for you, there are other options. There are coffee substitutes made from roasted carob, malted barley, chicory and even dried fruits and nuts. They have a rich flavour but can be a tad bitter. There are plenty to choose from on sale in health shops.

### Dandelion Coffee

One of the more popular coffee substitutes is dandelion coffee, made from roasted dandelion roots. Dandelion coffee is good for the liver and kidneys as well as digestion problems and is rich in anti-ageing materials. However, I have never found one I like and, personally, would rather have my favourite alternative to coffee, green tea.

### Green Tea

Green tea contains a tiny amount of caffeine but also an abundance of antioxidants so, as far as I'm concerned, this is a fantastic coffee substitute – and you don't get withdrawal symptoms!

Green tea originated in China 400 years ago and has been found to help protect against cancer and heart disease. According to a British study, published in 2000, it may also strengthen bones in post-menopausal women. The research found that women aged between sixty-five and seventy-five, who drank one cup of green tea daily, had higher bone density in their spines and thighs than those who didn't.

Scientific evidence from France has also shown that drinking green tea can help you lose weight. A study showed that obese women who drank green tea while on a diet lost three times as much weight as those who did not. It seems drinking green tea can boost your metabolic rate by as much as 4 per cent.

## White Tea

White tea is beginning to get an even better press than green tea. There isn't any scientific data at the time of writing, but it is well known that this much rarer tea is even richer in antioxidants than green tea. Traditionally, in Chinese medicine, white tea is used to detox and to strengthen the immune system.

It is the least processed form of tea because it is made from the first spring shoots of the plant, and is sweeter than green tea. If you can find it, it is well worth purchasing

## Rooibos

Rooibos is a very popular tea replacement that is completely caffeine-free. It is recognized by scientists for its ability to help with allergies because of its high flavonoid content. Japanese research has suggested that it may have a beneficial effect on some skin conditions and, in Britain, some animal herbalists recommend rooibos tea for calming excitable animals!

Whether you like it or not, rooibos contains enough free-radical scavengers to place it high on the anti-ageing shopping list.

## Ordinary Tea

I think ordinary 'builder's' tea is worth a mention here because of its benefits, as long as it's organic. The caffeine in tea has a different and less negative effect on the body compared to pure caffeine.

The amino acid theanine is found in all teas, and is a known relaxant. Having a cuppa may be as de-stressing as having a long soak in a hot bath. Theanine also *increases* GABA and dopamine, the brain chemicals that put you in a good mood, whereas caffeine *decreases* them.

Finally, if you love your cup of tea, give the teabag a good squeeze to increase the amount of flavonoids in it; this will help fight the free radicals in your cells and give you a good chance of ageing healthily and being wrinkle free. One or two organic cups a day, without milk and sugar, are a definite OK for this anti-ageing programme.

## Other Hot Drinks

Dandelion tea: helps drain the liver and gall bladder, so great for a detox
Nettle tea: stimulates the kidneys to release more water naturally, rich in calcium
Fruit teas: full of toxin-fighting antioxidants
Detox teas: liquorice, dandelion, fennel seed, parsley and turmeric all help to support the liver and the adrenals
Miso instant soup: sold in sachets and rich in dipicolinic acid for taking toxins out of the body safely

## Super Alcohol

I bet this heading grabbed your attention! Although there are plenty of reasons why alcohol is ageing, there also seem to be quite a few reasons why it isn't. Regular studies (probably funded by the wine producers) have shown that consuming small amounts of red wine can help prevent heart disease because it contains the potent antioxidant resveratrol, known to help stimulate enzymes that prevent cell death.

But, according to many anti-ageing experts, drinking alcohol causes a rapid rise in blood sugar and therefore inflammation, or oxidation, throughout the body. Mild dehydration will cause a

3 per cent drop in metabolism, resulting in ½ kilo of weight gain every six months.

As I like the odd glass of red wine myself, here's my solution. At any one time only drink a couple of *small* glasses of a good red wine such as Merlot, Cabernet Sauvignon or Pinot Noir for maximum flavonoids. Drink plenty of water in between the glasses as this will help put out the 'inflammation' the wine causes in the body as well as preventing dehydration. And always drink wine with food to avoid a rapid rise in blood sugar.

As far as any other alcoholic drink goes, again, moderation is the key to everything. Just try and drink the least sugary and yeasty options such as dry white wine, tequila or vodka. One of the biggest agers is stress, so if a little drink completely relaxes you, then it can't be doing that much harm can it?

## Super Soups

This chapter can't be finished without a mention of soups. As explained earlier, as liquid meals don't need much energy to digest, that energy can be used instead to keep your cells youthful. Home-made soups are easy to make, cheap and highly nutritious. They are filling and, especially in the winter, warming and will keep you going for hours.

You can make soups out of most of the vegetables in Super Foods by combining 4 cups of your favourite veg, along with 4 cups of vegetable stock and flavouring. Simmer for ten to twenty minutes and then blend.

Here are recipes for two summer and two winter soups using the very best of the antioxidant, anti-ageing vegetables. I have used cups as a measurement to make it simpler. Just use the same sized cup throughout the recipes.

## GAZPACHO

Serves 4
*1 small red onion, finely chopped*
*3–4 tomatoes, peeled and de-seeded*
*1 red pepper, de-seeded*
*1 cucumber, chopped*
*1–2 tablespoons cider vinegar*
*3 tablespoons olive oil*
*2 cloves garlic*
*½ can tomato juice*
*unrefined crystal or sea salt to taste*
*2 teaspoons vegetable stock or bouillon powder*
*2 spring onions*
*fresh parsley, basil, marjoram or thyme*

Purée or blend the chopped onions, tomatoes, half the red pepper and half the cucumber. Add the vinegar, olive oil, garlic, tomato juice, and seasoning to taste. Finely chop the spring onions, the rest of the cucumber and red pepper and fresh herbs and add to the top of the soup. Refrigerate. Delicious and cooling in the summer and quite filling. Add sunflower or sesame seeds instead of croutons if you need some crunch!

## SPINACH AND AVOCADO CHILLED SOUP

Serves 4
*500g spinach*
*flat-leafed parsley*
*ground almonds to thicken the soup*
*500ml vegetable stock*
*500ml quark or 'live' yogurt*
*2 ripe avocados, peeled and stoned*
*salt*
*dash of Tabasco*
*juice of 2 limes*

Chop off the spinach stalks, wash and place in a saucepan with a little water. Cover and cook for 5 minutes. Drain well and let it cool. Add the parsley, nuts and stock. Bring to the boil, cover and simmer for 10 minutes, stirring occasionally. Leave to cool then add the quark or yogurt. Purée and pour into a bowl. Purée the avocados with a little of the soup, then stir into the rest of the soup, and season. Cover and chill in fridge for 2 hours. To serve, add Tabasco and lime juice. This soup is absolutely delicious and very filling.

## CLEANSING WATERCRESS SOUP

Serves 4
*6 cups vegetable stock*
*6–8 spring onions, finely chopped*
*fresh herbs*
*2 sweet potatoes, peeled and sliced*
*4 bunches watercress, chopped*
*400ml milk or alternative milk*
*lemon or lime juice*
*salt*

Heat 1 cup of stock in a large saucepan. Add the spring onions and herbs, cover and simmer for 5 minutes. Add the potato and the rest of the stock to the saucepan, cover and simmer for another 20 minutes, until the potato is cooked. Add the watercress and simmer for 2 minutes. Turn off the heat and add the milk. Stir well and leave for 5 minutes. Blend until smooth and creamy. Re-heat, add lemon or lime juice and salt according to taste.

## RED PEPPER SOUP

Serves 4
*2 tablespoons olive oil*
*1 red onion, chopped*
*3 cloves garlic, finely chopped*

1 medium sweet potato, peeled and cubed
2 teaspoons paprika
½ teaspoon chilli powder
1 teaspoon cayenne pepper
2 tablespoons coriander, chopped
salt
2 cups shredded cabbage
2 cans tinned tomatoes
5 cups vegetable stock
1 tablespoon honey
1-2 fresh red chillies, diced and de-seeded
2 red peppers, de-seeded and diced
½ cup coconut milk

Heat the oil and fry the onion, garlic, potato, spices and coriander for 5 minutes. Season. Then add the cabbage, tomatoes, vegetable stock, honey and chillies. Simmer until the potato is cooked. In another saucepan, sauté the peppers in a little oil. Add them and the coconut milk to the soup. Adjust the seasoning. Purée when cool.

You should by now have a very clear idea of what foods, drinks and oils to use in your new anti-ageing regime. The next chapter will help you put it all together so you can decide which type of eating plan you want to follow.

# 6.

# Super Anti-Ageing Diet

I am now going to take you through four different anti-ageing 'diets' so you can pick one that best suits you and your lifestyle. These are the raw and living diet, the hunter-gatherer diet, the glycaemic index diet and the food-combining diet. The raw diet will suit vegetarians, vegans and anyone living in a sunny, light, warm climate. The hunter-gatherer diet will suit those who can't live without meat and fish but are happy to exclude all grains from their everyday meals. The glycaemic index diet is for anyone who wants to eat both animal products and grains. It is particularly good for people who suffer from raging blood-sugar levels or are on their way to insulin resistance. Finally, the food-combining diet will enable you to reap enormous health benefits whichever regime you choose.

Once you choose a plan you like, think of it more as a guide for life rather than a quick-fix diet. You may wish to try each different diet for a couple of weeks to see how your body responds. If you feel bloated, lethargic or constipated then it doesn't suit you. Don't forget that anything that is not mentioned here *can* be eaten provided it can be found in Super Foods on page 50.

The four suggested diets are followed by Eat for Life, which is my personal concoction of the best of all the aforementioned diets in one plan that suits my busy life and hopefully yours! All these regimes have been extensively researched in the anti-ageing field.

At the end of this chapter you will find a selection of Super Tips (page 124) to help you get the maximum health benefits from eating, whether you choose to follow one of the diets or not!

## Raw and Living Diet

This is the plan that makes the most sense to me when it comes to anti-ageing, but is also the one that is the most difficult to follow completely if you live in the UK and have any kind of a life outside home!

According to Brian R. Clement, founder of the Hippocrates Program and author of *Living Foods for Optimum Health*, the cells of the body degenerate, mutate and die because they are not fed properly. Unlike cooked, processed or animal foods, 'living' foods can supply the cells with the nutrients they need to grow and regenerate: vitamins, minerals and proteins as well as oxygen, enzymes and alkalinity. Regenerated cells are young cells.

There is, however, a slight difference between living and raw food. Living food is something that is 'alive' such as wheatgrass or alfalfa sprouts, raw food is something that hasn't been cooked but isn't necessarily still 'living': raw fish is an example. If you left a piece of raw fish on the kitchen counter, it would go off and smell. On the other hand, if you leave some seeds to soak overnight they carry on 'living' and sprout and would, if planted, grow. If a food cannot produce life because it is 'dead' then how can our cells produce more 'life' for us if we feed them with foods that have no vitality or energy? According to Clement, anyone who eats a diet of living foods automatically improves their health, mental aptitude, immunity and slows down their ageing process.

We are the only species on the planet that cooks and processes food and this is the reason, according to Clement, that we are malnourished in alkaline foods, enzymes, hormones and oxygen, all of which are essential for strong cells and a healthy, young immune system. 'No physical ailment known today cannot be arrested or improved with the Hippocrates Program,' he says.

The body defends itself against the ravages of free radicals with an army of antioxidants and enzymes that repair damaged cells and break the free radicals down into water and harmless oxygen. This process is interrupted when we eat *cooked* foods because cooking increases the number of free radicals and reduces the number of enzymes supplied to the body.

This is not a new theory. Microbiologist, Dr Paul Kouchakoff, carried out extensive research into the effect of cooked food on the body back in the 1930s. He discovered that every time cooked food is eaten, the body reacts as it would to an infection or a toxin by increasing its number of white blood cells in a process called leukocytosis. Highly processed foods such as white sugar, ham, vinegar and wine produce the most severe reaction. Animal products of any kind, but especially those cooked or processed, are therefore responsible for all those saggy bits on our bodies: folds around the mouth, flabby arms and cellulite-ridden thighs – all signs that our cells are ageing.

So, to revitalize and renew your body you should have a diet that excludes all cooked food and all animal foods. When we go back to nature and eat a diet rich in vegetables, fruits, seeds, nuts and grains we increase our chances of keeping cells clear of acidic debris which keeps the immune and digestive systems strong and functioning right to the end of old age.

If these claims are correct, then just think what living foods can do for the ageing process. I have met Brian Clement, who has eaten nothing but 'living' foods for several decades, and I can vouch for how young and clear-skinned he looks. My concern is that a raw, living-food diet is quite difficult to follow in a northern climate.

### WHY A RAW AND LIVING DIET IS ANTI-AGEING

- *The enzymes in living foods break down excess fat, leading to weight loss.*
- *Cooked, processed and artificial foods waste the immune system's energy.*
- *It keeps cellular energy high and acidity low.*
- *It slows ageing and improves mental agility.*
- *It boosts the body's immunity.*
- *The longer you do it, the more your body will detox and the younger and healthier you will become.*

Like all strict vegetarian or vegan diets, a living-food diet improves health and slows the ageing process by eliminating meat and dairy products. This de-clogs the veins and arteries and reduces the build up of protein deposits that over many years will have made the body highly acidic and, possibly, leached calcium out of the bones. This makes complete sense to me, but living without omega-3-rich fish does not.

I have, therefore, adapted the raw and living diet to one that can be more easily followed in a cold, dark climate such as the UK where most people find it hard to follow in the winter when they want to eat warming foods rather than salads. Dr Kouchakoff tested many foods that are usually excluded on this diet and found that if they were fresh, unrefined and not *over*heated (as in poached) they did not cause leukocytosis. Think un-browned, un-burnt foods. So oily fish is back on the menu, unless you want to be a complete purist.

## EASY WAY TO EAT A RAW AND LIVING DIET

- *Eliminate smoking, drinking, coffee, sugar, meat and dairy products as much as possible. You can include live yogurt and unpasteurized cheese and some oily fish.*
- *Aim for half to three quarters of your food being raw.*
- *Begin each meal with a large salad, raw vegetables or a juice.*
- *Have fresh fruit for dessert and for snacks, but no more than 15 per cent of your diet should come from fruit.*
- *Nuts and seeds should be soaked for 2 to 12 hours to release enzymes, or grind them into a fine powder.*
- *Have soaked nuts for breakfast with almond milk.*
- *Use tahini, hummus, spicy bean pinto, avocado, seaweed and other protein-rich foods instead of animal protein.*
- *Eliminate all processed food.*
- *Cut down on bread, unless it's made from sprouted grains, or use one of the recommended grains as a substitute.*
- *Add sea vegetables to your diet.*
- *Cut out all sugar.*

- *If you must cook: poach, steam or bake your food. Don't let it brown. For the sake of your health 'bin it if it's brown' is very good advice because of the free radicals produced.*
- *Do not fry food.*
- *Keep alcohol to a minimum and have it only occasionally and with meals.*
- *Cut out coffee and tea. An occasional cup is OK, but let it cool first.*
- *Herbal teas should be treated as 'cooked' foods. Allow them to cool down.*
- *Dried fruits are usually heat treated so only consume small amounts.*
- *Fresh olives are better than tinned or in a jar.*
- *Avoid large quantities of soya as it contains hormone disruptors.*

I consider 'live' yogurt and unpasteurized cheese made from raw milk to be pretty close to 'living', so I do still have a little animal protein on this plan. I can't quite stomach a green vegetable juice for breakfast, so go for the easy option by carrying on with my usual bowl of 'live' goat's yogurt with lots of living foods such as soaked wolfberries and bee pollen from the next chapter added to it. That could be why I haven't noticed the folds round my mouth improving!

It is extremely difficult to follow a raw and living diet completely in the UK, especially in the winter, but is possible. I still manage to eat a big, raw, living salad every day and start each meal with a raw vegetable juice, raw vegetables, alfalfa, or a rocket salad if I am in a restaurant. But if none of this resonates with you, maybe the hunter-gatherer diet will. If you can't live without meat but can live without grains, this is the one for you.

# The Hunter-Gatherer Diet

Human beings are omnivores in that we eat both plant and animal foods. Dr Loren Cordain, from the Department of Health and Exercise Science at Colorado State University, is widely acknowledged as a leading expert on the natural diet of our Paleolithic relatives. He has published numerous studies proving the dramatic health benefits of eating a diet we had been following for thousands of years.

Before we learned to sow grains, our ancestors gathered fruits, roots, nuts, seeds, herbs, eggs and vegetables and ate anything they could hunt: birds, wild boar and fish. Every bit of the animal was eaten including the internal organs and brain and they even ate insects and worms. In fact we still have a unique enzyme in our bodies, which is just for breaking down insects! Their diet was naturally rich in omega-3, antioxidants and nutrients that protected them from most of the diseases we die from today.

Today, more than 70 per cent of our dietary calories come from foods that our Paleolithic ancestors rarely, if ever, ate. The result is epidemic levels of cardiovascular disease, cancer, diabetes, osteoporosis, arthritis, gastrointestinal disease and more, because, according to Dr Cordain, the human body just didn't have time to evolve to cope with this change.

I think there's another reason why carbs and starches are blamed for everything from gut problems to insulin resistance and weight gain. We eat too much of them for the amount of energy we're using and most of them – especially refined carbohydrates – are full of additives, preservatives, salt and sugar. They are as far from their natural state as it's possible to get.

If you are going to eat meat it should be organic, free of chemicals, growth hormones, artificial additives and preservatives, just as it was thousands of years ago. This will ensure the foods you consume are as close to nature as possible and still contain the nutrients that help you live longer. It does, however, make this plan a pricier one to follow.

Here is a list of foods that are *not* allowed on the hunter-gatherer diet. It is very similar to the GI diet, except that here you can't eat certain grains or lentils. There is also a short summary of the foods you *can* eat.

## DO NOT EAT THE FOLLOWING

- *All grains: particularly bread, pasta, noodles, wheat*
- *Beans/peas: string beans, kidney beans, lentils, peas, peanuts*
- *Potatoes or sweet potatoes*
- *Cashews*
- *Dairy products*
- *Salt*

## YOU CAN EAT

- *Meat*
- *Offal*
- *Poultry*
- *Fish*
- *Eggs*
- *Fruit*
- *Nuts (except cashews)*
- *Seeds*
- *All other vegetables, including salad, and roots other than potatoes or sweet potatoes*

If you decide to follow the food-combining plan, the hunter-gatherer diet is relatively easy to follow. But you do need to like your flesh!

## The Glycaemic Index Diet

The glycaemic index (GI) is a measure of how quickly a food raises blood-sugar levels, which depends on the amount of carbohydrate it contains. The higher a food is on the GI, the faster it releases sugar into the bloodstream and the more it affects your blood-sugar levels.

A *gradual* rise in blood sugar, on the other hand, and therefore of insulin, have proven benefits for health. This plan offers you plenty of high-protein and low-carb starches, but also eliminates a lot of starchy vegetables such as cooked carrots and a few popular anti-ageing fruits. It is essential reading for anyone with diabetes in the family or terrible energy fluctuations.

As discussed earlier in the section on hormones (page 28), only two hormones increase with age and one is insulin. Starchy carbs release large quantities of insulin into the body and the more your diet contains fast-releasing carbohydrates such as pastries, biscuits and even Cornflakes, the more insulin is produced and the more your blood-sugar levels fluctuate. Over time, the insulin receptors and the pancreas get exhausted from the constant demands on them and, at worst, insulin resistance sets in. At best, the weight piles on.

Insulin resistance is affected by our age, the menopause, smoking and, most importantly, diet. Women suffer more because they naturally have lower levels of serotonin. These feel-good chemicals decrease even more during menstrual cycles. Later in life fluctuating hormones may cause us to reach for a nice sugary chocolate bar to boost our blood-sugar and serotonin levels, but it has the opposite effect. Yes, we get a nice serotonin high, but this is swiftly followed by a blood-sugar low and, in the long term, more fat around the middle!

From the carbohydrates you eat, your body absorbs simple sugars into the bloodstream which it will then turn into glucose. The glucose is converted to glycogen to be stored in your muscles and liver to give you energy. However, if the glycogen stores are full and there is still more glucose coming in, the excess will be converted straight to triglycerides – fat to you and me.

Not only that, but sugary starches and foods cause glycation, which, according to dermatologist Dr Nicholas Perricone, is the main cause of leathery skin. You don't have to be diabetic to experience an inflammatory response from sugar; a healthy body is also damaged by sugar. According to Dr Perricone, when foods rapidly convert to sugar in the bloodstream as carbs high on the index do, they cause browning, or glycation, of the protein in your tissues. In your skin it causes damage to collagen and that means deep wrinkles, which Perricone refers to as cross-linking.

The skin of someone whose collagen has been cross-linked from years of eating carbs and sugars does not snap back and smooth out like a young person's, because the wrinkles are due to the sugar molecules attaching themselves to the collagen, making the fibres stiff and inflexible. This bonding between sugar and collagen generates a huge number of free radicals leading to more inflammation, so your skin looks like tanned hide.

If you want young, non-leathery skin, want to lose weight and balance your blood-sugar levels, it is important to become aware of the foods that release sugars very fast. The list on page 117 is of the *bad* carbs and starches.

Some of the fruits and vegetables in this bad carbs list will surprise you, because they appeared in the anti-ageing Super Fruit and Super Veg section (pages 53 and 57). They do, however, release sugar much faster than other fruits and vegetables so should be considered worthy of exclusion *if* you are seriously worried about your blood-sugar levels. A baked potato is not an unhealthy food but it contains a lot of carbohydrate and does take a lot of digesting. Use your common sense and don't worry too much about the bad carbs in the second half of this list; you can eat them occasionally. Try to eliminate all the truly bad carbs in the first half, because they have no part in an anti-ageing plan.

Anything not on this list is fine to eat or drink. If they are in Super Foods go ahead and have anything from there. If you have raging blood-sugar levels, go easy on the fruits and cooked root vegetables, as they are high in natural sugars and could make you feel drowsy after consuming them. Just listen to your body. If you feel like a nap forty minutes after eating something, you've eaten the wrong food for your body!

## BAD CARBS

*Very high in sugar and with no health benefits*
- Sugar
- Cakes
- Pastry
- White Pasta
- White Rice
- Crisps
- Chocolate
- Bagels
- Shredded Wheat
- Weetabix
- Glucose
- Alcohol
- Biscuits
- White Bread
- Popcorn
- French Fries
- Croissants
- Sweets
- Soft Drinks
- Cornflakes
- Sports Drinks
- Mashed Potato

*High in sugars but with some health benefits*
- Baked Potato
- Maize
- Sweet Potato
- Tea
- Orange Juice
- Black Eyed Beans
- Melon
- Grapes
- Cooked Carrots

- *Milk*
- *Corn*
- *Parsnips*
- *Dried Fruit*
- *Red Kidney Beans*
- *Pineapple*
- *Banana*
- *Honey*

Be aware of sauces, pickles and ketchup etc. They are all loaded with sugar, as is chewing gum, even if it's artificially sweetened.

## The Food-Combining Diet

Food combining helps many people who have digestive problems in a matter of days. It also helps keep you young. It works because the load on the digestive organs is less, the food is digested and absorbed better and more nutrients get to the cells. The body produces less fermenting gas and toxins, so many people with food allergies do better as well. Correct food combining produces an increase in energy levels, because the body doesn't need as much energy for digestion.

When you combine foods properly you may well also see excess pounds and slack skin start disappearing. Most people who practise good food combining lose real fat as opposed to water. Your digestion works better, so your body doesn't require as much water to flush out the cells it would otherwise need to get that cheese sandwich moving through your gut! Bloating will be a thing of the past, and you will probably eat less because you are absorbing your nutrients better.

A fourteenth century Italian nobleman and writer lived to age 102 on two meals a day totalling 12 ounces of food and 14 ounces of grape juice. He began at thirty-five when his health fell apart after a lifetime of overindulgence. However, I don't know how young he *looked* on all that glycation-causing grape juice! Whether he lived to such a ripe old age purely because of food combining, or not, following this kind of regime takes *less* energy away from the digestive system, which gives the body *more* energy for constant cleansing and regeneration.

Different foods are digested differently. Starchy foods require an alkaline environment and are digested, initially, in the mouth. Protein foods require an acidic environment and are digested in the stomach. Acids and akalines neutralize each other, and that's when the trouble starts, especially as people get older. If you eat starch and protein together the digestion is put under stress. A meal such as steak and chips can take a very long time to get through the system, causing havoc as it goes. Undigested food ferments and produces gas, bloating and often constipation.

## TEN EASY STEPS TO FOOD COMBINING

1 Don't eat protein and starch at the same meal. For example, no meat and potatoes, cheese and bread, baked potato with grated cheese. Well, you won't be eating those anyway, will you?
2 Don't eat two proteins from different sources at the same time, for example, cheese and fish.
3 You can eat two different types of fish at one meal, prawns as a starter, salmon as a main course.
4 Eat nuts separately from your main meal.
5 Don't eat starch and fruit together. The stomach digests the sugar first, causing it to ferment and creating acid, which destroys the enzymes needed for digesting the starch. So, no fruit and cereal for breakfast.
6 Eat melons separately from other foods. As with all fruits, they don't combine well with any other food, but as they are digested very quickly they can be eaten as a starter.
7 Eat all other fruit on an empty stomach.
8 Pulses are both protein and starch. They can be mixed with either protein or starch foods.
9 Don't eat milk or milk products with other foods. I find this one tricky as I like live yogurt with curry and in smoothies.

10  Skip pudding. Eaten after a heavy meal it will just lie on the stomach fermenting away!

It isn't at all difficult to follow this plan. Try it for at least a week and see how much better you feel. Less digestion equals more energy so it's worth a try.

So that's four different diets to consider. One may have popped right out at you as the perfect one for your lifestyle and taste buds. But if which one to follow confuses you, try my simple Eat for Life Master Plan which encompasses all four regimes but highlights only the healthiest of the anti-ageing foods from each.

## Eat for Life

This section is my own personal eating plan incorporating the best of the preceding diets, and one that suits both my life and taste buds! It won't suit everyone, but it is a simple reminder of what you should eat lots of and what you should avoid for maximum energy and a youthful skin. I eat as much raw and living food as possible, love oily fish, eat good meat occasionally, consume low-carb starches and use food-combining principles wherever possible. If you have similar tastes to me, use the lists in Super Foods and incorporate these pointers.

### Vegetables

Make the main part of your meal raw vegetables or steamed if you have to (see list on page 54). The anti-ageing, green vegetables should take up half your plate, along with a handful of alfalfa sprouts. Go easy on parsnips, pumpkin, corn, potato, sweet potato and cooked carrots as they are all very high in starch and convert to sugar rapidly.

## Fruits

Blueberries, cranberries, strawberries, raspberries, loganberries and blackberries are the top anti-ageing fruits. Eat melon, grapes, pineapple, banana and dried fruit in moderation, as they are all very high in natural sugars. Try to eat fruit on an empty stomach and wait an hour before eating something else for perfect food combining.

## Fish

Eat three to four portions a week of omega-3-rich oily fish such as salmon, mackerel, sardines and tuna. All fish is good for you, but make sure to check the list on page 61 for the most and least beneficial.

Poach or bake fish rather than frying or roasting. The less brown it is, the less it is oxidized and the fewer free radicals are produced. Even better if you like sushi – the fish will be raw!

If you want the health benefits of oily fish but can't stand the taste you can do what I do when I'm away from home and make sure to take an EPA 1000mg fish-oil capsule with every meal.

## Meat

Reduce your consumption of red meat as much as possible, but if you like to eat meat make sure it is free range, grass fed and/or organically raised. If you always have a Sunday roast, have a small portion of meat with *six* anti-ageing veg instead of meat and two veg! Again, check the list on page 62 for the healthiest and the unhealthiest options.

## Vegetarian Options

Eggs and all pulses are complete proteins and can be eaten instead of meat or fish. If you are prone to swinging blood-sugar levels, eat black-eyed beans and red kidney beans in moderation because they are high in starch. I am addicted to tahini, spicy bean pinto and hummus. These can all be found in good health stores, middle-eastern shops or supermarkets.

## Dairy Alternatives

Eat any of the suggestions on page 66 in strict moderation. Sometimes a rocket salad needs a bit of Parmesan to liven it up, but it's worth remembering that all cheese whether unpasteurized or produced by a goat is still high in fat and can add inches if consumed in excess.

I do, however, usually have live goat's yogurt for breakfast, along with the foods I recommend in the next chapter because, as a practitioner, I believe it is important to give the adrenals protein first thing to help them function better. Live yogurt also encourages good bowel bacteria as well as being high in calcium.

Almond milk is a good drink to get into making if you really love a glass of milk or want milk in your smoothie. Almonds are loaded with calcium but are low-fat nuts. Learn how to make it on page 67.

## Grains

My favourite grain, high in protein and low in starch, is quinoa, and instead of bread I eat Dr Karg organic seeded spelt crispbreads (found in Waitrose or health stores) or sprouted grains. There are plenty of other grain options for you on page 68.

## Nuts and Seeds

I have listed the best anti-ageing nuts and seeds on pages 69 and 71, but for maximum anti-ageing benefits, soak them for a minimum of two hours, preferably overnight, or grind them. This makes them easier to digest and releases more enzyme activity, so they deliver more nutrition.

I start every day with a tablespoon of soaked flaxseeds/linseeds. They are nature's HRT because of the high phytoestrogen content – and they keep my bowels very regular!

## Sea Vegetables

Incorporate as many from the list on page 76 as possible because sea vegetables provide you with all the magnesium, calcium, potassium and sodium your body needs, as well as a large amount of iodine to support the thyroid, naturally and safely. I sprinkle nori flakes on my food three to four times a week to make sure I'm getting enough.

## Oils

I use coconut or olive oil for cooking and a tasteless flaxseed oil, mixed with a little olive oil, for salads.

## Salt

If you need salt, use crystal or unrefined sea salt. It should be pink or grey not white.

## Drinks

Try and cut down on coffee and builder's tea as much as you possibly can. Coffee seems to be public enemy number one among all anti-ageing experts. Replace it with green or white tea for the fantastic antioxidant properties.

Don't forget your body needs 2 litres of water a day if it's going to age well. That's just one glass an hour.

TOP TIP FOR MEALTIMES

*Start every meal with something raw and living, if you can, to get all that enzyme activity going to protect you from any free radicals the food produces. The best of the anti-ageing bunch is a handful of living nutrient-dense alfalfa sprouts popped on top of your meal and eaten before anything else. You can even take a carton with you to work or when you go out to eat. Just tell people it helps your digestion!*

### RAW and LIVING OPTIONS

*A shot of wheatgrass juice with a juiced orange or tangerine*

*A vegetable juice made up from any of the vegetables suggested
    in Super Foods or Super Drinks on pages 54 and 99*

*Melon*

*Fruit juice – wait an hour if you are following this with protein*

*Raw vegetable batons with a dip such as hummus*

*Half an avocado with lemon juice and one of the recommended
    oils*

*Rocket, spinach or watercress salad*

### MAIN MEALS

*You have plenty to choose from in Super Foods but if you are at
home and want a super anti-ageing meal, try my favourite salad
and dressing (see page 227), along with some oily fish or a
warming, high-protein grain such as quinoa.*

A word about vinegar. Lemon or lime juice are both better for
anti-ageing as they increase the alkalinity in the body, so use them
in preference to vinegar whenever you can. But if you must have
vinegar, make it organic, cider vinegar not the over-fermented,
yeasty vinegars such as balsamic.

At every main meal, try and eat a small green salad first and
then go on to your favourite protein. If you *have* to eat starch with
this meal, make it one of the grains from the list on page 68. Again,
choose a protein-rich grain towards the top rather than the grains
that contain gluten at the bottom.

 SUPER TIPS

*Start the day with hot water and freshly squeezed lemon juice
    to kick-start your liver.*

*Eat the most watery food first, and then the next most watery.*

*Eat less: the smaller the meal, the less time it takes your body to
    digest and the more energy you have.*

*In lab experiments, mice lived twice as long when their calorie
    intake was halved.*

*The long-living inhabitants of Okinawa eat 17–40 per cent fewer calories than we do in the West. They have more centenarians than any other population.*

*Have one main meal a day and two snacks if you can.*

*Stop eating when you are 80 per cent full. Wait half an hour and you probably won't feel hungry any more. You will have reduced your calorie intake by 20–30 per cent so can expect to live a long and youthful life!*

*Have a liquid-only day once a week to give your digestion a really good rest. You can make natural healthy soups or smoothies.*

*Eat at least one third less food than you are used to.*

*Skip a meal a couple of times a week.*

*Don't snack.*

*Don't eat anything after 7 p.m.*

*Don't drink anything while eating, because the liquids dilute the enzymes and stop your stomach from doing its job properly.*

*Chew all food almost to a liquid. Drink your foods and eat your drinks! Foods that aren't chewed properly will pass through your body without depositing all those nutrients.*

*If you find yourself in a restaurant and can't possibly do without a pasta dish, or a similar naughty, just make sure you have something fatty with it. If you have butter, olive oil or Parmesan cheese, the fat will slow down the absorption of the starchy carbs, and slows down the rapid blood-sugar conversion and that glycation.*

You now know how to Eat for Life and you will hopefully master and incorporate the suggestions into your daily life. In the next chapter, we look at six Super Supplements that are, with the exception of one, anti-ageing 'foods' rather than pills, that you can easily add to a smoothie, yogurt, cereals, drinks and even soups.

# 7.

# Super Supplements

There are so many anti-ageing supplements it would take another book to cover them all. The conclusion I have reached as a practitioner is that an awful lot of people, especially as they get older, don't absorb supplements as easily as the same nutrients found in natural food. So, with one exception – a homocysteine-lowering supplement – the supplements I'm recommending – fish oils, wolfberries, spirulina, bee pollen and maca – are all living foods, as opposed to chemically produced supplements. However many vegetables and juices you consume there is still a chance you may need higher amounts of certain nutrients than the food can provide, so here are my own personal favourite anti-agers to add to your food. Every single one of them is something I take every day, no matter how well I'm eating. They're my insurance policy and I really feel a difference without them.

The first three – fish oils, wolfberries and spirulina – are 'foods' that will supply you with every vitamin, mineral, amino acid, and nutrient you need. If you are vegetarian, vegan or following the raw living diet, these three are essential. For anyone else, they can all replace expensive supplements in a more absorbable form.

## Fish Oils

I'm sure you know by now why EPA fish oils are here, right up front. As you have seen, their high omega-3 content, easily broken down by the body, makes them an essential addition to your daily diet, unless you are eating oily fish 5 times a day, 5 times a week. Even if you eat oily fish daily, as I do, fish oil capsules make absolutely sure you are getting a minimum daily dose in an absorbable, toxin-free form.

Just to recap, many scientists believe that the major reason for the high incidence of heart disease, hypertension, diabetes, obesity, premature ageing, and some cancers, is the imbalance between our intake of omega-6 and omega-3 fatty acids. Our hunter-gatherer ancestors ate these fats in a ratio of 1:1, but today we eat something like a ratio of 20:1.

Omega-3 is found in great concentrations in flaxseed oil, flax-seeds, walnuts, hazelnuts and pecans and in the plankton fish eat. But the fatty acids that are most beneficial, when it comes to ageing, come directly from fatty fish and fish oils (EPA and DHA). The alpha-linolenic acid in seeds and nuts has to be converted to these two components by the body and the older we get, the harder it gets. There is still a very important place in any anti-ageing diet for plant foods that produce omega-3, especially for vegetarians and vegans. But to get these precious fats straight to where they are needed: to every cell in the body, every gland, every organ, there is nothing better than EPA fish-oil capsules.

Danish doctors discovered the benefits of EPA and DHA in the seventies when they noticed that the Greenland Eskimos had an exceptionally low incidence of heart disease and arthritis, despite their exceptionally high-fat diet. Seal blubber and oily fish are both exceptionally high in EPA and DHA.

The human brain just hoovers up DHA, the most effective of the omega-3 fatty acids. It needs high levels to avoid low serotonin levels, which can cause depression, SAD, moods and forgetfulness. A high intake of fish oils has been linked to significant improvements in memory, moods and mental problems as well as lowering the risk of developing ageing-diseases such as Alzheimer's. Nothing cheers my clients up more during the winter months than a couple of fish-oil capsules a day.

Professor Michael Crawford, DHA research expert from the Institute of Brain Chemistry and Human Nutrition, at London Metropolitan University, says that 'DHA is as important to the brain as calcium is to the bones.'

Omega-3 fatty acids help to produce the prostaglandin 3 series which has been shown to reduce the inflammation of arthritis, blood pressure and heart disease as well as improving cholesterol levels, hormone production, metabolism, nerve transmission and gut function. In fact, everything! Especially plumped-up, young-looking skin.

DMAE, found in high quantities in fish-oil capsules, is a powerful antioxidant that stimulates nerve function and causes the muscles to contract and tighten under the skin. If you want younger skin and can't face eating oily fish on a daily basis, this is the supplement for you. Take it even if you do eat omega-3-rich foods daily; it will serve as an insurance policy as your body simply can't get enough of it. As I mentioned in the previous chapter you can always take one 1000mg capsule with every non-oily-fish meal for maximum skin benefits.

## FISH-OIL NUTRIENTS

- *Vitamin A for healthy eyes*
- *Omega-3 for a healthy heart, joints and brain*
- *Zinc to boost the immune system*
- *DMAE for plumped-up skin*
- *Nucleotides for healthy DNA*

You should buy the best-quality fish oils you can afford. Low-quality fish oils may be unstable and contain chemicals and toxins. High-quality oils are processed and packaged carefully and are stabilized with vitamin E. Look out for fish oils that are packaged in a lightproof tub or box and make sure they are rich in EPA and DHA – not all of them are. Pure fish oil that is in liquid form is probably the best quality, but, personally, I can't stomach it off a spoon, it reminds me too much of my mother forcing cod liver oil down me as a child – for which I am now eternally grateful!

Cod liver oils and fish oils are not the same. Cod liver oil is extracted from cod liver, and is a rich source of vitamins A and D, as well as a little EPA and DHA, but not enough. The liver is also where any toxins are stored, which could be passed on to you. Fish oils are extracted from the *body* of the fatty fish and, although they contain less A and D than cod liver oil, they contain much higher levels of EPA and DHA.

Fish oils are safe to take and have not, to date, been found to cause any problems. However, I have seen warnings about taking them if you are on any kind of blood thinner so I recommend you check with your doctor first if you are on any kind of medication.

It is also a good idea to take extra vitamin E (200mg) with fish oils as the oils can lower the amount available in your body. Anyway, any extra vitamin E can only help your skin improve even more.

I recommend at least 2 × 1000mg capsules a day for my clients. It is safe to take up to 4000mg a day, but no more. It's been proved that there is no extra benefit in taking much more, so you might as well save your money.

Any of the health benefits from 2000mg a day should be seen within a few weeks, but it may take a few months for degenerative diseases such as arthritis and atherosclerosis (high blood pressure) to improve.

## Wolfberries

Wolfberries come from wild bushes that grow in China and are also known as goji berries (which means wolf in Chinese) or the Lycium barbarum fruit. They are known as 'happy' berries because it is said that a handful of them will keep you jolly for the rest of the day. Not only that, but these little red, raisin-like fruits are associated with longevity and, unlike ginseng, large amounts can be eaten continuously over a long and happy life. And there's more!

These delicious little berries are so beneficial to your health you can use them instead of the following supplements:

WOLFBERRIES REPLACE

- *Antioxidants A, C and E*
- *Vitamins $B_1$, $B_2$ and $B_6$*
- *21 trace minerals including: zinc, iron, copper, calcium and selenium*

- *Echinacea*
- *St John's wort*
- *Sleeping pills*
- *Milk thistle*
- *Blood-sugar supplements*

Wolfberries also contain eighteen different amino acids, including the eight essential ones such as isoleucine and tryptophan. They also contain leucine, an essential amino acid for anti-ageing which helps you burn fat and build muscle.

Here are just a few of the ageing conditions a handful of wolfberries a day will improve:

Immune system: the berries contain polysaccharides that strengthen the immune system. The same polysaccharides stimulate the human growth hormone, the *youth* hormone that decreases body fat and firms muscle.

Fat burning: Lycium barbarum has been tested as an anti-obesity drug. Patients were given 30g each morning and afternoon, made into tea. Most patients lost significant weight. I certainly have!

Eyesight: wolfberries have the highest content of beta-carotene on the earth, which can dramatically improve eyesight.

Liver: wolfberries improve liver function, protect the liver and encourage new hepatic cells to grow.

Blood pressure: eating wolfberries regularly helps maintain healthy blood pressure whether it needs to come down or go up!

Cholesterol: these berries have been used to reduce cholesterol in clinical studies.

Blood-sugar levels: they are used in China to treat diabetes and maintain blood-sugar levels. I use them in my clinic for blood-sugar problems with great success.

Longevity: in Asia wolfberries are famed as a giver of longevity. A gentleman called Li Qing Yuen is said to have lived to 252 years, a fact authenticated by both Eastern and Western scholars, due to eating a soup of wolfberry fruit every day *from* when he was fifty years old!

Anti-ageing: it is a powerful antioxidant fruit that prevents and reverses free-radical damage. It also maintains normal cell growth and improves DNA restoration and repair.

For the elderly: twenty elderly people were given wolfberry extract once a day for three weeks. More than 67 per cent of the patients' T-cell functions tripled and their white-cell activity doubled. Their spirits and optimism increased significantly and there was a 95 per cent improvement in appetite and sleep. More than a third recovered their sexual function.

You can use wolfberries to make tea, soup, stew and even wine! You can chew them like raisins, or soak them, like I do, to release all the enzymes and nutrients. The recommended daily amount is 8–30g a day.

For my clients on the run, I advise them to take a bag of wolf-berries to work and munch on them instead of chocolate. It works, they snack less, lose weight, have improved blood-sugar levels and love them! They are also great for kids. What an easy way to get antioxidants into children. You can't eat too many of them *unless* you are suffering from diarrhoea (in which case you shouldn't be eating any soft fruit!) or if a practitioner in Chinese medicine, for example an acupuncturist, has told you that you have 'dampness' or spleen deficiency. Always check if in doubt.

TOP TIP

> *Soak a bowl of wolfberries overnight for maximum nutrient and enzyme release. You can then add a couple of tablespoons to your breakfast.*

## Spirulina

Spirulina is my 'must have' when I am away from home because it gives me everything my body needs in just six small tablets, and keeps me going when I'm working hard. It is an absolute must for the over fifties as an anti-ager, energy booster and immune supporter. Although it is in pill or powder form, I consider this one of nature's most natural and nutritious super foods.

Spirulina is the botanical name of a blue-green alga, and algae are known in the anti-ageing world for promoting cellular regeneration as well as providing all the vital elements that are missing from ordinary land-based foods. Algae help convert toxic waste material into harmless substances, provide protection from free radicals and supply a balanced profile of vitamins, minerals and essential amino acids.

Spirulina is also known as an 'energy' food because scientists have discovered that when it's fresh it is a powerhouse that stores and converts enormous quantities of solar power into green chlorophyll, blue phycocyanin and orange carotenoids, the natural pigments that give spirulina its deep green colour. It gives anyone who takes it regularly extra vitality and optimum health.

## Main Nutrients

**Protein**: spirulina contains all twenty-two amino acids, including the essential eight, so it is a source of complete protein in a more absorbable form than that found in many animal products. Very useful for vegetarians, vegans and anyone following the raw and living diet.

**B$_{12}$**: it is one of the few plant sources of vitamin B$_{12}$ providing more than twice the amount found in liver, making it essential for vegetarians and vegans and anyone who doesn't eat offal, as well as anyone following the raw and living diet. Vitamin B$_{12}$ absorption decreases with age so spirulina can benefit anyone who wants more energy.

**Phycocyanin**: a blue antioxidant that strengthens the body's resistance by pursuing free radicals that damage and age the body.

**Polysaccharides**: increase the body's antibody production and infection-fighting T cells.

**Gamma-linolenic acid** (GLA): an essential fatty acid that can help control the symptoms of PMS, particularly painful breasts and fluctuating hormones and many other conditions. It protects the skin against sunlight and dehydration and boosts blood circulation.

**Iron**: fifty-eight times richer in iron than spinach, safer for the thyroid and easier to absorb than in supplement form.
**Beta-carotene**: twenty-five times richer than carrots.
**Chlorophyll**: twice as rich as barley and wheatgrass.

If that isn't enough to convince you, this little super food is also packed full of other nutrients and benefits.

## Spirulina Helps

**Weight loss**: taken between meals spirulina helps boost energy levels, suppresses the appetite and provides the body with nutrients. It is part of any weight-loss regime I put my clients on.
**Stamina and endurance**: greatly improve.
**Recovering from illness**: it provides the body with a good source of protein and essential minerals and vitamins to aid recovery.
**For the elderly**: in older people, spirulina helps maintain a healthy digestion. This is essential for anyone who isn't eating properly, or can't, because it provides the body with the nutrients it needs. Many older people don't eat enough, have restricted diets or suffer from poor digestion. They may have low energy and be undernourished. This is an excellent supplement because it is 60 per cent protein and easy to digest. Anyone suffering from arthritis or raised cholesterol can also use spirulina as a safe replacement for meat.
**Skin health**: spirulina can also be used externally as well as internally. The high beta-carotene content will help improve the elasticity of the skin, as well as the health of the eyes. It is rich in vitamin E, selenium and zinc, which protect the skin from free radicals. The chlorophyll it provides helps take oxygen into the skin's cells. The high content of tyrosine, a natural amino acid, slows down the ageing process of the cells and helps protect the skin against sunburn.
**Bone health**: gram for gram, spirulina contains more calcium and magnesium than most other foods.

Look out for a top quality, 100 per cent natural spirulina that has been grown without herbicides or pesticides. Hawaiian spirulina is considered to be the most potent and pure in the world.

Take the tablets or capsules with or after meals. Swallow them whole with water. Six tablets will give you the minimum daily dose of 3g. Or take a heaped teaspoon of powder, which you can add to smoothies or a fruit juice. The most suitable juice is citric and sweet, such as orange juice.

There are other algae on sale, such as chlorella and super algae that will work just as well to support your health and help the ageing process. They are all extremely beneficial but none of us has a limitless budget so I have suggested the algae I regularly use and feel the benefits from. By all means try any alternative you come across, as they will do you just as much good.

## Bee Pollen

This is also true for bee pollen. There are some very powerful honeys, royal jelly and other products made by bees available. They are all extremely useful for protecting our health and preventing ageing. I just happen to use bee pollen because I like the taste.

If you want to make sure of getting your essential anti-ageing B vitamins every day, a teaspoon of this lovely stuff will deliver all you need plus a whole lot more. Bee pollen is renowned for its anti-ageing properties because it can rejuvenate the cells, stimulate the organs and glands, give you more energy and help you to live longer.

Pollen is the fine dust collected as honeybees land on flower petals to harvest plant nectar and is brought back to the hive in tiny pouches on the back of the bees' legs. The granules are trapped as the bees enter the hive, without harming them. So when you eat bee pollen you are basically eating pure plant nutrients.

Honeybee pollen contains more than 5,000 enzymes and co-enzymes, many more than *any* other food. It is so powerful it can protect against radiation, X-rays, radiotherapy and environmental pollutants. It can also produce a visible improvement in the appearance of ageing skin. According to research in Europe, pollen is the richest source of protein in nature containing five to seven times more protein than cheese, meat or eggs, as well as being a valuable source of $B_{12}$ and the other Bs essential in later life, including choline and folic acid. Pollen is the only known food that has every essential nutrient needed by the body for perfect health, often referred to as nature's most complete food. It contains all twenty-eight minerals found in the body and lecithin which protects the nervous system from ageing and flushes out fat. From Hippocrates to Pythagoras, the fathers of Western medicine have extolled its virtues for its healing properties and as a secret weapon against old age.

Bee pollen is renowned for its anti-ageing properties. It is a source of vitamins E and P which keep skin youthful. It prevents premature ageing of the cells and promotes the growth of new tissue. It contains nucleic acids which smooth away wrinkles and stimulate the blood supply to all skin cells. Because of its high content of vitamins and protein, the collagen and elastin of the skin will strengthen and look younger.

Apart from all the benefits to the skin bee pollen can bring you, there are a whole host of ageing conditions that it can also help: loss of libido, high blood pressure, depression, low immunity, stress, fatigue, high cholesterol. It also promotes the health of the brain, the liver, the pancreas, the thyroid and the heart.

And more good news for anyone suffering from menopausal symptoms, bee pollen can help alleviate – fatigue, hormone headaches, hot flushes, urinary incontinence.

The effects take a minimum of three months to become apparent, but I must share with you one huge success I have had with bee pollen. I have always had a weak bladder and was well on the road to stress incontinence, until I started using bee pollen daily. My bladder became stronger within a couple of weeks and I rarely suffer from that terrible urge to go. I have no idea why or how it works – but it does!

Take 1–2 teaspoons daily. These little golden, coloured granules are very easy to eat but can cause a heavy stomach, bloating or diarrhoea. So start with only a few and build up very slowly till you can have a teaspoon without any side effects. You can sprinkle it on yogurt, cereal or bread or take it straight off the spoon. I sprinkle a teaspoon on my breakfast bowl of yogurt and if I need a quick boost of energy in the afternoon I put a teaspoon *under* my tongue so it is absorbed straight into the bloodstream more quickly. It is another fantastic all-rounder if you have an elderly or sick relative.

I have listed where I get my bee pollen at the back of the book in the Resources section on page 234, but you can try any health shop or the internet for yours.

## Maca

Sometimes known as Peruvian ginseng, maca is a sweet brown powder that comes from the roots of a hardy cruciferous vegetable, which grows high in the Andes in a cold, oxygen-poor environment. It is a member of the cabbage, broccoli and Brussels sprout family but, unlike its English relatives, because the soil of this area is extremely rich in minerals, the plant is too. Native Peruvians have used maca for several thousand years as a food and medicine to improve fertility, libido and energy.

More importantly, maca is an adaptogen, which is essential for anti-ageing as it helps the body cope with and reduce stress. Since 1947 medical and scientific research has been carried out on adaptogens in various parts of the world, but has recently become available to us in the West. Explaining the effects of the adaptogens is difficult, since they affect each of us differently.

If you are mentally exhausted or physically tired, adaptogens will help you feel more energetic, vitalized and full of zest for life. But they are not normal stimulants. If you are stressed, emotionally drained or just not coping with life, adaptogens will help you relax and make life easier to cope with. But they are not tranquillizers.

In other words, adaptogens help your body adapt to whatever is upsetting its equilibrium, without suppressing it. Rather than address a specific symptom, adaptogens improve the *whole* system, helping the body to adapt and return to normal balance.

Maca is rich in all the minerals you need for optimum health, as well as B vitamins. But most importantly for an ageing body and ageing hormone production, it contains four alkaloids that have been shown to nourish the endocrine glands. Dr Gloria Chacon de Popovici is a biologist from South America who, in 1960, isolated the four alkaloids responsible for the medicinal effects of maca. Her research revealed that they acted on the hypothalamus and pituitary gland, which work together to regulate the other glands, including the adrenals, thyroid, ovaries and testes, by releasing higher levels of precursor hormones (hormones that produce more hormones).

Maca revitalizes the middle-aged and elderly both mentally and physically as well as helping with fertility, libido and maintaining menopausal hormonal balance. It is useful for treating chronic fatigue as well as stress, depression and immune weakness. But, most importantly, it is a safe, natural alternative to HRT, alleviating so many of my clients' symptoms like hot flushes, vaginal dryness, depression, fatigue and osteoporosis, that it has become a must for any woman of a certain age.

Take 1–2 heaped teaspoons of maca daily. It can be mixed into a smoothie or with apple, cranberry or pineapple juice and put in a blender for a few seconds. It can be sprinkled on cereals, added to soup or you can, like I do, mix it into a bowl of live yogurt, along with the wolfberries and bee pollen. It is best to take it in the morning for sustained energy throughout the day.

So these are all the anti-ageing supplements in 'food' form that I recommend. You don't need to take all or any of them to age healthily, but they will certainly help. Maca is a true supplement and a totally essential one if you have heart disease, dementia or Alzheimer's in the family.

## Homocysteine-Lowering Supplements

Homocysteine is a toxic protein found in the blood that can damage the arteries including the arteries in the brain as well as the heart. Homocysteine is linked to more than fifty diseases and, according to Patrick Holford, nutritionist and author of *The H Factor*, there are seven thousand published papers to date to prove this. At least three out of four people die from preventable diseases. The big five are: heart attacks, strokes, cancer, diabetes and Alzheimer's disease. According to Holford, you should be able to add ten–twenty years to your life if you change your diet and take a homocysteine-lowering supplement that includes folic acid $B_{12}$, $B_6$ and TMG.

Homocysteine is ageing in every way. If you expose the cells that line arteries throughout the body to homocysteine, they age more rapidly and are more prone to damage and premature death. The main cause of this damage is free-radical oxidation. High homocysteine levels dramatically increase free-radical oxidation and the damage caused by it. Researchers at the University of Bergen in Norway found that there was a strong relation between homocysteine and all causes of death. If homocysteine levels are reduced, the cells age more slowly and vitality increases.

In the mid-1990s a study was published in the *Journal of the American Medical Association* proving that homocysteine was more important than cholesterol in predicting heart attacks and that at least one in five people with a history of heart disease had high homocysteine levels. Holford predicts that within the next ten years checking for homocysteine will become a routine part of a medical check-up as common as checking cholesterol levels and blood pressure is today. I have just seen a client whose doctor had measured his homocysteine levels, so it is obviously becoming more well known.

The reason a homocysteine-lowering supplement is so important for the health of your brain, apart from keeping your arteries unfurred, is the high content of tri-methyl glycine (TMG) present in any decent supplement. TMG is a natural polysaccharide extracted from sugar beet (also produced as betaine) which promotes antioxidants that protect you against homocysteine damage in the brain. TMG also helps prevent depression. It is essential for the healthy production of the neurotransmitters that help produce hormones for a happy, healthy brain.

## HOMOCYSTEINE-LOWERING SUPPLEMENT BENEFITS

- *Improved mood, memory and mental clarity*
- *Improved liver function*
- *Better hair, skin and nails*
- *Increased energy*
- *Better sleep*
- *Raised glutathione levels, which slow the ageing process*
- *Dramatic reduction in the risk of heart disease, strokes, cancer and Alzheimer's disease*

If you value your heart and brain health, get this one supplement, especially if you are over fifty or have heart disease or Alzheimer's in the family. You can have your homocysteine levels tested by getting in touch with your doctor or sending away for a blood test from a laboratory.

You will find various homocysteine-lowering supplements in your local health store or on-line, but do first check that they contain the ingredients mentioned, especially TMG or betaine with $B_{12}$, folic acid and zinc.

## Immun'Age: Boost Your Immunity and Banish Ageing

Here is an extra anti-ageing food supplement which has served me very well during particularly exhausting and stressful periods. You might like to try it a couple of times a year for a huge boost to your immunity and skin health. It is called Immun'Age and is receiving unprecedented praise in the press as an anti-ageing miracle, but it's not cheap! It is a powder, made from 100 per cent fermented papaya preparation (FPP) which promises to: 'Boost energy levels, return the glow of a healthy complexion and protect against loss of elasticity and the onset of wrinkles.' It is claimed to be used by celebs from Hollywood to Holyhead and is receiving rave reviews from them too.

Immun'Age is a specialized nutritional supplement backed by more than thirty scientific studies to date. It has been used in Japan for decades and is also very popular in France, where they know a thing or two about skin care. The process begins by slowly fermenting fresh, ripe papayas in a natural process that takes several months. The fermented papaya is then dried and ground into a fine powder. This phytonutrient-rich powder can then be sprinkled in the mouth, dissolved (preferably under the tongue) and swallowed. This is another 'must have' supplement for me to take when I travel because it is so easy to carry around and use.

Scientific studies have found this preparation is able to fight two of the main reasons we get old – oxidative stress and immune-system decline. Researchers who studied the properties of papaya found that when they combined papaya with specific yeasts and traditional Japanese fermentation techniques, FPP was born. You will remember how beneficial this fermentation technique is in other Japanese foods, such as miso and tempeh.

FPP was then subjected to rigorous scientific studies to prove that it was a superior antioxidant, a powerful immune-system booster and one of Japan's secrets to a long, healthy life.

Oxidative damage is the number-one factor in facial ageing, caused by free-radical damage. If oxidative stress is prevented, the skin is likely to keep its youthful appearance for longer. FPP contains unique and powerful antioxidants that neutralize this damage. It does this by affecting superoxide dismutase (SOD) and glutathione peroxidase (GPX), the pathways that eliminate free radicals from the system. SOD is sadly missing in most of the antioxidants I have written about so far, which makes this anti-ager an antioxidant with a plus. Since ageing is largely determined by how well our bodies can fight oxidative damage, using this product may well slow down the ageing clock.

The immune system starts to decline with age mainly because our white blood cells become less efficient in keeping viruses and bacteria from infecting us – much like us, they just get too tired to fight and let the invaders in. FPP helps the macrophages (the white cells that eat bacteria, viral particles and free-radical fragments) work faster and ingest more. Scientists have also discovered that FPP increases the production of interleukin which plays an important part in wound healing and keeping minor infections from becoming major infections. It also boosts the activity of natural killer cells (white blood cells) which can help protect us against cancer.

Immun'Age costs £40 for a month's supply, but you only need it for three to four months a year as a general booster. I spent five days over the summer, camping at a festival, not sleeping much, getting chilled to the bone and generally leading a lifestyle that would batter the most robust immune system! I took this supplement twice a day for the whole time and came home with nothing worse than a cold that went more quickly than any cold I have ever had.

So that's a quick summary of my favourite supplements. They are worth considering, but are by no means essential, apart from maybe the homocysteine-lowering supplement. I use them all and reap their benefits daily. You can find out where to buy the brands I use in the Resources section on page 233, but there are plenty of alternative sources on-line or through a health store if you prefer.

# 8.

# Super Bod

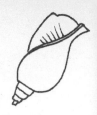

This is a romp round the body to help you get the maximum out of each part in your fight against ageing. Starting from the top, we begin with hair which is one of the first things to look dull and lacklustre as we get older.

## Super Hair

Falling oestrogen levels can result in thinning hair as well as dull, coarse and greying hair: that so-called natural process of ageing. According to John Mason, president of the Institute of Trichologists in London, one of the other main reasons for thinning hair in women is a sluggish thyroid, which needs iodine to help it function properly.

Here are a couple of quick tips to improve the condition of your hair.

TOP TIP

*Although I haven't yet found something that completely prevents greying hair, wheatgrass is supposed to be extremely helpful. It takes a full twenty-one days for wheatgrass to take its full effect so be more patient than I have been!*

TOP TIP

*Replace your normal hair tint with an organic, natural one if you can. Recent research shows that long-term use of hair dye, for more than a decade, on dark brown or black hair in particular, may be increasing the risk of non-Hodgkins lymphoma (and God knows what else) by up to four times.*

## Loss of Hair

To encourage growth, the spirulina mentioned in the last chapter will certainly help. It has made my already very thick and fast-growing hair (and nails), grow even more quickly, which means the grey needs retouching every month instead of the usual six weeks. An unexpected bonus/disadvantage! Although there is a decent amount of iodine in spirulina, you may like to add a kelp supplement or sea vegetables to your regime to help support the thyroid which will, in turn, strengthen your hair and nails.

Nettle tea is also very good for encouraging hair growth as it's high in vitamin C and natural silicone, which helps protect and strengthen the hair shaft. Eat your sprouts — any of the living sprouts (as well as cucumber) are rich in silica which strengthens hair, nails and skin.

## A Natural Conditioner

Egg yolks are brilliant for the hair because they are full of lecithin and all the amino acids that help cells grow stronger. Beat a couple of egg yolks and use them instead of your usual shampoo. They clean, condition and encourage healthy, thick hair growth.

## Dry Hair

Soak elderflower teabags in warm water and then use the water to rinse your hair after washing. Elderflowers are cleansing and help restore natural moisture.

Increasing essential fatty acids omega-3 and 6 will help even more. Remember that EFAs are a natural moisturizer and prevent the skin and scalp from becoming dry and flaky.

## Greasy Hair

Lemon juice is ideal as a final rinse because the citric acid helps cut down the fat your hair holds onto. Cider vinegar is also wonderful for naturally restoring the pH balance of your hair and scalp. As a final hair rinse, add two dessertspoons to 500ml of water and pour over the hair and scalp. This will get rid of dandruff *and* add natural highlights!

### Glossy Hair

For soft, glossy locks try half a teaspoon of glycerine mixed with half a cup of rosewater and comb it through dry or wet hair. Leave it to dry and brush well.

## Super Eyes

I haven't tried all these suggestions for improving my ever deteriorating eyesight, but I can pass on a few tips that have helped temporarily if not permanently!

TOP TIPS

*Stop smoking – all those thousands of toxic chemicals go straight into your eyes. (That's why mine are so bad – years of smoking before I knew better.)*

*Wear sunglasses in the sun.*

*Drink 2 litres of water a day.*

*Follow the anti-ageing diet and increase your consumption of:*

*Antioxidant-rich berries such as blueberries which protect the eye blood vessels.*

*Beta-carotene-rich carrots – after three weeks of drinking juiced carrots daily, I had to have my eyes re-tested because my eyesight had improved between the eye test and the glasses being made. The optometrist couldn't believe her eyes.*

*Spirulina and wolfberries both have one of the highest levels of beta-carotene in the world, so you can try one of those instead of carrots.*

*Lutein and zeaxanthin can help improve eye health because they act as potent free-radical scavengers for the retina. Both are found in dark green foods such as spinach and broccoli and also in eggs. There is a spray you can buy to take orally,* that contains eye nutrients such as lutein, bilberry and gingko biloba. This is available from reputable health stores or on-line.

Exercise every day to help oxygenated, fresh blood reach your eyes' cells.

Look after your liver and your liver will look after your eyes: read the section on the liver (page 155) and eat wolfberries daily – your bloodshot eyes, bags and puffiness should vanish.

Apply castor oil to clean your eyelashes: it will help them grow thicker and longer. Why do they get sparser and thinner with age?

Quick fix: green tea teabags soaked in hot water, chilled in a freezer then popped on the eyes, will help their appearance. The antioxidants in the tea reduce swelling and should put the sparkle back into the windows of your soul.

Eye tests: please have your eyes tested regularly, because the optometrist can discover a lot more than failing eyesight. Glaucoma, cataracts, diabetes, cholesterol build up, can all be diagnosed by looking at the iris.

If you work at a computer take a break every thirty minutes and rest your eyes. Looking into the distance for a couple of seconds as often as possible while working on-screen will also help. Your eye is a muscle and, like any other, needs exercising. Encouraging it to focus away from the screen regularly will keep it more flexible and help you avoid eyestrain. As hunter-gatherers we developed our long-distance vision, so the muscles are at their most relaxed when we use them for looking into the distance.

## Super Teeth

We have thirty-two teeth, if we're lucky, and we need to look after them if we are going to avoid wearing dentures. Another joyful part of growing older is that the supporting tissues around the teeth start weakening. According to my dentist, people lose teeth and end up having to wear dentures because of just two things:

gum disease or tooth decay. The anti-ageing diet will prevent the tooth decay and cleaning your teeth properly will take care of the gum disease. Teeth can also give our age away if they look yellow and the gums are receding and unhealthy. Here are some top teeth tips.

TOP TIPS

*Only sugar can penetrate a tooth's strong enamel coating. Give it up.*

*Sugary fruit and dried fruit can be almost as detrimental to your teeth's health as sweets.*

*The thousands of chemicals, smoke and tar in cigarettes make the teeth yellow and cause bad breath.*

*Bad breath can also be caused by ear, nose or throat problems. If you have bad breath and have ruled out bacteria or a poor digestion, see an ENT consultant. Gargling with warm, salty water can also help.*

*Coffee and tea stain the teeth: only drink 1–2 cups a day.*

*Not flossing could kill you. Yes, I thought that might grab your attention. Christine Toye, my dental hygienist, confirms that flossing daily and using an electric toothbrush can reduce the risk of heart disease because the bacteria that form between your teeth and gums, if not removed, can get into the bloodstream and circulate to the heart. It is only likely to happen if your gums are bleeding – but the risk is a real risk, she says, especially among the middle-aged. Floss before you brush your teeth because you are less likely to be too tired and go off to bed without doing it and the brushing will take away all the debris you have just dislodged. Debris becomes plaque if it's not removed.*

*Massage your gums to remove toxins and get the blood flowing. Always brush your gums as well as your teeth and brush behind as well as in front of your teeth.*

*See a dentist every six months to a year.*

*See a hygienist every three months to a year.*

*If your teeth look really old and yellow, consider having them
whitened. Some whitening products are available over the
counter, although I have only found one that works in
America. Large department stores can bleach them in your
lunch hour. Visit your dentist for the best advice. It's not
cheap, it's not 'natural' but it's well worth considering if you
feel unhappy every time you smile.*

*The antioxidant effect of vitamin C appears to increase healing
in the gums. Any fruit rich in vitamin C will help.*

## Super Ears

For most of us the main problem we are likely to suffer from as
we get older, apart from failing hearing, is a more frequent build
up of earwax. I think the message about *not* sticking cotton-wool
buds down your ears on a daily basis and poking about has got
through. Syringing also doesn't seem as popular among the medical
profession as it used to be. Most nurses, doctors and specialists
now agree it is much safer to soften the wax naturally by using
a little warmed olive oil every day for at least three weeks. I
was incredibly ill after I had my ears syringed for the first time
in twenty years. It could have been totally unrelated, but I'll
never have it done again. It's the old-fashioned way for me from
now on.

Chronic ear infections are associated with an over-consumption
of wheat, milk, corn, egg, yeast, soy and sugar. The anti-ageing
diet will have eliminated most of these and lessen your chance of
suffering from frequent ear problems.

If you use a Walkman or iPod, do keep the volume down, and
if you love loud music and go to live concerts or clubs frequently
you might decide, surreptitiously, that it's time to put a little cotton
wool in your ears to protect the ear drums. Such wisdom comes
with age!

## Super Bones

Osteoporosis affects one in three women and is responsible for over 200,000 broken bones a year and forty deaths a day in the UK alone. It is often thought of as a silent disease because people don't know they have it until it's too late. Bones begin to weaken after thirty and by middle age they could have become fragile and brittle, with the wrists, hips and spine particularly at risk.

### What Causes Osteoporosis

A poor diet in youth can weaken the bones in later life and before. High-protein diets, fizzy drinks, yo-yo dieting and even over-exercising have been linked to an increase in the number of young women showing bone-density results comparable to people thirty years their senior. An excess of protein can cause a complete imbalance in the body's mineral deposits and produce an over-acidity that can further weaken bones. Soft, fizzy drinks are loaded with phosphorus which, in excess, drags calcium out of the bones.

The National Osteoporosis Society reports an increase in the disease among young women, particularly those who are underweight and those who have suffered anorexia.

As you have already seen the body stops producing oestrogen at the menopause and this is the hormone essential for good bone health.

### What Prevents Osteoporosis

A diet high in Super Foods and enough exercise, but not too much, is key. Exercise at least three times a week for a minimum of 20 minutes. Anything that puts your joints under stress has been found in scientific studies to be the best exercise to help prevent osteoporosis because it increases bone density. Gentle jogging is the most effective, but doesn't suit everyone.

## Super Breasts

Breast cancer is the single biggest killer of women in this country causing a thousand deaths a month – the highest mortality rate in the world. However, it is now generally accepted that more than a third of cancer deaths worldwide are caused by modifiable risk factors. Dr Sara Miller, specialist in Integrative Medicine and Senior Doctor at Bristol Cancer Help Centre, confirms that certain lifestyle changes may reduce women's breast cancer risk. 'We advise women to follow a healthy lifestyle by eating a diet high in fruit and vegetables, drinking less alcohol, avoiding cigarettes, exercising regularly and reducing stress.'

The anti-ageing diet (page 108) will help protect you against most types of cancer, but there are a few other things you should take on board if you are concerned about breast cancer.

### REDUCE YOUR RISK OF BREAST CANCER

- *Try giving up smoking for good.*
- *Exercise on a regular basis, aim for three to four hours a week – more tips on page 189.*
- *Take up pastimes such as yoga or tai chi to reduce your stress levels.*
- *Eliminate unwanted oestrogen and other hormones by having less tap water, red meat and dairy products. They may contain stored hormones or pesticides.*
- *Limit consumption of alcohol to no more than two alcoholic drinks a week.*
- *Keep to the anti-ageing diet for its anti-cancer nutrients.*
- *Lose weight and keep it off. Excess weight has been associated with an increased incidence of breast cancer, according to the World Health Organisation.*
- *Avoid excessive amounts of soya (see page 63).*
- *Carry out regular self-examination checks.*
- *Visit your GP if you are at all concerned about changes in your breasts.*

## Super Lungs

Breathing is something we do without thinking, sixteen times a minute, taking in around 13,500 litres of air a day. But most of us are not breathing deeply enough to fill our cells with an essential vitamin – vitamin O for oxygen! Without it we have no life and at the very least no energy. Breathing is directly connected to how you age. You need oxygen to take nutrient-rich blood all around the body and to keep your skin healthy and young.

There is a breathing exercise called pranayama described on page 206. It is a yogic form of breathing that increases your intake of oxygen to help keep your skin young, increase energy levels, sharpen your brain and give you strong lungs.

For now, just consciously start taking deep, purposeful breaths, right down to your stomach instead of shallow breathing from the top of your lungs.

## Super Heart

They say you are only as old as your arteries. After forty many people experience up to a 20 per cent decline in their maximum heart rate during exercise because the heart becomes less responsive. Blood vessel's narrow, arterial walls stiffen and there can be a 20–25 per cent increase in blood pressure by middle age. Women have 15 per cent less cholesterol than men pre-menopause, but post-menopause it has risen to exactly the same level.

However, some of the risk factors of heart disease happen a lot earlier. A cardiologist told me recently that 90 per cent of GIs killed in Vietnam were found in post mortem to have hardened arteries and they were barely past twenty. Furring of the arteries starts early, however fit you are. We need to concentrate on our heart's health, not only to live, but because all the major arteries to and from the heart also flow to all our major organs, including the brain. To avoid dementia we need clean, clear arteries so the best nutrient-filled blood is taken all over the body to keep us young.

TOP TIPS TO AVOID HEART DISEASE

*Eat more pulses which are rich in folic acid, which helps depress homocysteine, the amino acid that promotes clogged arteries and heart disease.*

*Eat less red meat: vegetarians are 30 per cent less likely than meat eaters to die of heart disease.*

*Make sure you get lots of antioxidants which protect your arteries and heart as well as your skin and brain.*

*Eat a clove of fresh garlic a day; research confirms that garlic can reduce cholesterol.*

*So can lecithin. Lecithin helps prevent fats from accumulating on the walls of the arteries.*

*Reduce your intake of saturated fats: cheese, lard, suet, bacon, fatty meats and hydrogenated fats such as margarines and spreads.*

*Don't add salt to your food – a diet high in salt is a prime cause of high blood pressure – a major cause of heart disease and strokes.*

*Increase your EFAs – omega-3 has been shown to lower triglycerides and cholesterol levels and prevent hardening of the arteries. It helps maintain the elasticity of artery walls, prevents blood clotting and reduces blood pressure.*

*After a heart attack a person eating oily fish three times a week halves the risk of another.*

*Research suggests that drinking green tea may protect against heart disease.*

*Reduce stress. Exercise releases endorphins as well as strengthening your heart. The heart is a muscle as well as an organ and needs exercising. The endorphin releases from exercise will help you relax. Dance your socks off round the kitchen for 20 minutes or take the dog for a walk. Do anything that is a stress buster. There are lots more tips on stress busting on page 202.*

*Regular yoga or tai chi sessions have been found to reduce the heart rate and blood pressure dramatically in three months.*

*Sleep apnoea, which affects four in every thousand snorers, has also been linked to a twenty-fold increase in the risk of a heart attack. See your GP if you suffer from sleep apnoea.*

*Increase potassium in your diet. A recent study discovered that people with least potassium in their diet were one and a half times more likely to have a stroke.*

*Eat more:*

*bananas – rich source of potassium as well as providing folic acid*

*apricots and figs – high in potassium*

*leafy dark green veg – provides potassium and folic acid*

*Smoking starves the arteries of oxygen – give up.*

## Super Tum

The digestive tract is one long tube from the mouth to the colon. Much like our muscles, the digestive system ages and weakens as we get older. Most people will start having digestive problems between forty-five and fifty-five as the body's ability to produce digestive enzymes reduces by half. Middle-age spread is very common among people with a poor digestion.

 TOP TUM TIPS

*Bloating: the very best thing to do is* not *eat. Fasting is the ultimate form of cleansing, even if you only miss a couple of meals, and is great for curing a bloated stomach.*

*Chew your food very, very well, a minimum of twenty times if you can manage it. The more you chew, the better the body absorbs the nutrients.*

*Try digestive enzymes or make sure you eat raw alfalfa sprouts before every meal. If your body isn't producing enough digestive enzymes a supplement will really help. I took them with me all over the world on a two-month trip (a bit difficult to take sprouts) and didn't have one day of bloating or constipation. Look for one that contains hydrochloric acid or brome-*

lain, as these are the enzymes older bodies have more difficulty producing.

Don't eat if you're stressed. Stress affects the digestion big time. It affects the gut, causes food intolerances, digestive problems and toxic build up. Have a smoothie, or a liquid meal instead.

Don't drink liquid with your meals – it interferes with the digestion.

Rest for a minimum of five minutes after eating. If you want a relaxed digestion and an end to bloating, sit quietly, or lie down, at the end of your meal and do nothing.

Drink hot water and lemon first thing in the morning to wake up your digestion. It really works and makes your body alkaline instead of acidic.

If your stomach muscles are slack and un-toned, like most of ours are at this age, you will find a recommended exercise on page 199 to help firm up your abs as well as the rest of your body.

## Super Bowels

The colon may not be the largest organ of elimination, but it is the most important. Like many other practitioners, I believe a healthy body can't stay healthy if toxicity stays in the gut instead of being evacuated regularly.

The colon is about six feet long and should be about two inches in diameter. However, by middle age, after years of consuming hard-to-digest food, sugar and antibiotics, that tube may be full of mucoid plaque slowing the peristalsis (movement) right down. Constipation and other bowel problems are caused by stress, a poor diet and a lack of fluid. Don't forget the colon needs plenty of water to help push the waste through and out.

It is normal to go to the loo two or more times a day – just see how often your cat or dog goes! Food transit time should take less than twenty-four hours so no more than two or three meals are in the gut at a time. Your lunch today should be pushing out yesterday's lunch. The trouble is, most people I see are going once a day, if they're lucky, and think it is normal.

If the digestion in the stomach and ability to absorb in the colon isn't working properly food just doesn't get broken down, and the nutrients don't get absorbed and taken to where they are needed. Food ends up dumped in the colon where it just sits and rots. The result is bloating, gas and sometimes an enormous pot belly. Many people with almost normal body-fat readings have enormous guts simply because they are carrying around up to nine meals' worth of undigested food and kilos of putrefying bacteria.

On the anti-ageing diet, your bowel should work a lot better, but if it doesn't here is one top tip that never fails, and you will be getting a huge surge of nature's HRT at the same time.

 TOP TIP

*Put a tablespoon of golden flaxseeds in a glass last thing at night and, as they swell quite a bit, make sure there is plenty of water to more than cover them. The seeds are full of zinc as well as vitamin E and omega-3 so none of that goodness is wasted if you drink the water along with the seeds. In the morning the seeds will be nice and soft and gelatinous so they don't just rush through your intestines, but go very slowly, gently cleaning your colon like a broom.*

*Take them every day.*

One of my elderly clients had suffered from chronic constipation for five years and would be in such pain that she was forced to use laxatives. After just four days of eating soaked flaxseeds, she started going to the loo, naturally, every morning for the first time in years. Another client had not had a regular bowel movement since giving up cigarettes. Her body missed the nicotine trigger. She, too, said the soaked flaxseeds changed her life – and her bowels – for ever.

There are other products, such as psyllium husks, that really help a sluggish bowel, but soaked flaxseeds have so many other health benefits that they are my favourite cure-all. However, if you suffer from diverticulosis or any other serious colon condition, please *only* drink the water the seeds have been soaked in as the little seeds can get stuck in the pockets of the gut. If in any doubt, always check with an expert.

There are also plenty of products that replace bad bacteria in the bowel with good bacteria. Eating lots of raw and 'live' foods will certainly help the good guys proliferate, but if you feel you need a little extra help, look for a colon supporter that contains lactobacillus and oligosaccharides that encourage the growth of friendly bacteria.

One final word, if you are wondering what a perfect, healthy poo should *look* like – a pale, brown, big sausage, smooth and soft means a happy, healthy colon and a happy, healthy body! It will happen with the anti-ageing diet and the soaked flaxseeds. Promise.

## Super Liver

Although the liver is very fragile, it can renew itself almost entirely. It can be reduced by up to 90 per cent and still regenerate itself, given the right conditions, in just six weeks. I call the liver the body's chemical factory because every single thing that is taken into your body, unless it is injected or taken rectally, passes through it. It filters more than a litre of blood every minute, removing bacteria and toxins from circulation.

Liver stagnation and the need for detoxification usually occur after an excess of toxins or food, or both. Christmas is a prime example. Rich, fatty food, sugar and alcohol encourage the poor old liver to become swollen and sluggish and we feel 'liverish'.

### SIGNS OF A LIVER IN NEED OF A DETOX

- *Dark circles under eyes*
- *Spots*
- *Itchy skin*
- *Age spots*
- *Sallow skin*
- *Poor digestion*

- *Bloating*
- *Weight gain around abdomen*
- *Constipation*
- *IBS*
- *Fluid retention*
- *Headaches*
- *Foggy brain*
- *Allergies*
- *Hot palms or feet*
- *Unstable blood-sugar levels*

## What To Do

Give yourself permission not to eat. You probably won't want much food, so this is a perfect opportunity for a liver-flush juice (page 98) or just plenty of water, vegetable juices or fruit smoothies, or just hot water and lemon juice.

If you want to eat, make it plenty of fresh, raw or steamed vegetables, especially cruciferous veg such as broccoli, Brussels sprouts, cabbage, kale and cauliflower because of their high glucosinolate content that helps the liver detox. I wonder if that's why Brussels sprouts evolved as such an important accompaniment to the big Christmas feast?

Brown rice is considered the food of the liver in Chinese medicine, so make sure to have a small portion the morning after the night before.

Have your last meal of the day early, and get to bed before midnight, so your liver has nothing else to do during its regeneration cycle, from 11 p.m. to 3 a.m.

The majority of any alcohol has to be metabolized in the liver; give it a rest for a few days if you feel liverish.

### LIVER HELPERS

- *Nettle tea*
- *Dandelion tea*
- *Garlic*

- *Fresh ginger*
- *Turmeric*
- *Onions*
- *Radishes*
- *Wolfberries*
- *Lecithin*
- *Seeds and nut oils*
- *Olive oil*
- *Flaxseeds*
- *Beetroot*
- *Carrots*
- *Chicory*
- *Watercress*
- *Brazil nuts*
- *Citrus fruits*

And finally, milk thistle has been used as a traditional liver tonic for centuries to heal, protect and regenerate it. It is the perfect herb to take the morning after the night before in tincture or pill form.

## Super Thighs

All older women complain about their thighs and their cellulite, wobbly flesh or fat. Unless we're prepared to work as hard as Madonna, it is all a very depressing prospect. I think of those knobbly bits of puckered flesh – that also appear on the arms – as *toxic* fat, not just fat. Fat cells love toxins and chemicals and stash them away in places like the back of our thighs to protect the more important organs. Just look at youngsters who have perfect bodies but cellulite on their thighs – they're usually smokers living on junk food. So cutting out all toxins will certainly help.

Apart from diet, there are a few things we can do to improve the appearance of our thighs and arms. The right type of exercise is key, as well as skin brushing and massage. There are plenty of suggestions coming up. Meanwhile, here are a few cellulite-busting tips.

## CELLULITE BUSTERS

- *Don't drink fizzy drinks, even water. The bubbles bloat the cells and encourage cellulite.*
- *Try a seaweed wrap. Beauty salons promise immediate results after an hour of being covered in a seaweed mask, wrapped up in a heated blanket and left to sweat all those toxins out. It does work, but a course is recommended for best results.*
- *Manual lymphatic drainage (MLD) is a very gentle massage, which will stimulate the lymphatic system to drain and eliminate toxins. This has proved very successful, with a course recommended for best results.*
- *Regular aromatherapy massage also helps break down those fatty cells.*
- *Self-massage can also help the circulation, so have a look at the massage on page 180 and do it regularly.*
- *If you have a power shower, blast the areas of cellulite using circular movements.*
- *End your shower on a cool to cold blast to really get the lymph moving.*

## Super Lymph

The lymphatic system is like the guttering of the body, where all the debris gathers. It removes foreign cells and debris and eventually dumps them into the blood to be broken down and eliminated. It is a secondary circulatory system, running alongside the blood but, unlike blood, it has no pump of its own and relies on a little help to get it going. Every time we breathe or move we are helping 3 litres of lymph a day to circulate through the lymph vessels, into the nodes and out into the blood. But when the system gets blocked by an infection or overloaded by excessive toxins things can start going wrong. The congested lymph nodes don't drain properly, the circulation slows down and the cells don't get enough nourishment. The tissues will react according to where the lymph is blocked in the body, so if the lymph nodes in the head and neck are congested, your complexion can look dull, tired, old and flabby. Water retention is a major sign of blocked lymph.

Here are some tips on how to get your lymph moving so you look youthful, vibrant and get rid of those lumpy bits on your thighs and arms.

### LYMPH MOVERS

- *You can increase lymph flow by twenty times simply by breathing deeply.*
- *Skin brush daily before bathing or showering: this is explained in full on page 225.*
- *Alternate hot and cold water in the shower, to boost the lymph.*
- *Exercise daily for twenty minutes, walking will do. It will increase the lymph's movement by 100 per cent. Walking up and down hill will really get the lymph moving.*
- *Bounce on a mini-trampoline – a rebounder – for five to ten minutes a day. Bouncing works with the earth's gravity so when you get to the top of a bounce, you are weightless for a split second. When you get to the bottom of the bounce, gravity is increased by two or three times which really gets the lymph pumping.*
- *Bounce up and down in a swimming pool, or in the sea.*
- *Treat yourself to a regular massage.*
- *Consider an annual course of 'spring cleaning' – manual lymphatic drainage.*
- *Cut down on stress in your life. Stress restricts the flow of every blood vessel in the body.*

## Super Bladder

Incontinence is something that affects up to 20 per cent of older women, but is something few of us want to talk about or admit to, despite the enormous displays of incontinence pads on sale in chemists'! There are many different types including: stress incontinence, mixed incontinence and urge incontinence. The most common is stress urinary incontinence, accounting for nearly half of all cases.

**Stress urinary incontinence**: urine leaks when sneezing, coughing, laughing or straining. It is common in women after childbirth when their pelvic-floor muscles are weakened.
**Mixed urinary incontinence**: the same as stress incontinence with the added aggravation of a need to wee urgently.
**Urge urinary incontinence**: the accidental leakage of urine shortly after a very sudden and intense need to wee. It usually occurs after the age of sixty, but I suffered from forty-something onwards, especially if I came in from the cold, desperate to pee. I could barely make it to the loo on time!

Another bladder problem is recurring cystitis or other urinary tract infections. As many as one in four women suffer from these at some time in their lives. The most common cause is E. coli germs originating in the bowel which get transferred to the bladder if you don't wipe your bottom carefully! Some women also suffer from recurring or interstitial cystitis because their partners keep reinfecting them.

The best advice I can give you is as follows:

Always wipe your bottom from front to back
Always wee after intercourse
Avoid constipation and take in plenty of healthy bacteria in the form of live yogurt, a pre- or probiotic drink or supplement
Take aloe vera juice which is an anti-inflammatory – 1 dessertspoon twice a day
Drink a *minimum* of 2 litres of water a day
Avoid all acid or citrus fruits such as lemons, oranges, tomatoes, kiwis, etc.
Avoid alcohol, particularly white wine, champagne and brandy because of their acidity
Cranberry juice (make sure it's sugar free) contains proanthocyani-

dins which help prevent E. coli from sticking to the bladder wall but it can make symptoms worse in some people with interstitial cystitis so always take advice

Limit coffee and sugar – which you should be doing anyway!

When you have an attack take a teaspoon of bicarbonate of soda each hour to make urine more alkaline

There is also a condition known as overactive bladder: a frequent and urgent need to empty your bladder, when it isn't yet full. I think I've been suffering from that all my life, and always put it down to having a small bladder.

There are a few things you can do to help a weak bladder instead of seeking surgical or medical intervention. But of course, do see a doctor if it is causing you severe problems.

## What To Do For a Weak Bladder

Pelvic-floor muscle exercises strengthen and re-train the pelvic floor and sphincter muscles. Your doctor, physiotherapist, yoga or Pilates teacher or fitness instructor, is the best person to check that you are doing it properly. But it is something you need to do for the rest of your life. Every time you go to the loo: tense your pelvic muscles and stop the flow of urine for a few seconds before allowing it to flow again. This will strengthen your pelvic-floor muscles.

Try to lose weight: excessive weight will add pressure to the bladder. Definitely stop smoking. Limit caffeine and alcohol intake: this is one of the most helpful pieces of advice I have ever been given. A gynaecologist I once worked with explained that coffee or an alcoholic drink is as irritating as cactus spikes to an already unstable bladder. That certainly helped me.

Take bee pollen. I mentioned on page 135 how much this natural food helped me. I rarely have an uncontrollable urge nowadays, unless I have stopped for a coffee when out shopping.

Don't skimp on your water intake – it is essential for properly functioning kidneys, as well as the rest of your body, and does not act as either a diuretic or a cactus spike. Your bladder will get used to it, just make sure the water is at room temperature and not too cold.

## Super Feet

After the age of forty-ish, a lifetime of pretty but ill-fitting shoes will have taken their toll on our feet. According to podiatrist, Pauline Caldwell, bunions, in-growing toenails, corns and callouses are all a result of years of squashing our feet into narrow shoes. As middle age approaches, if you let the weight pile on, there can be extra pressure on the feet causing dropped arches. Obesity can also cause cracked heels that may be so bad they bleed.

As the feet are the furthest away from your head, the older you get, the more difficult it is to look at them or after them! A tummy might be in the way, your eyesight fails, or you are just not flexible enough to reach them.

Having a nice pedicure at the local beauty salon doesn't quite cut it once the feet start playing up. Pardon the pun. I now go and get my curling and in-growing toenails cut properly by a state registered chiropodist. A regular visit is part of my anti-ageing regime and keeps my feet in tiptop condition. Anyone over forty should go for regular treatment to a qualified specialist, especially if they are suffering from systemic diseases such as diabetes. It is best to find a state registered chiropodist or podiatrist who will be able to remove callouses, sort out your corns and cut toenails properly.

So that's a quick trip around what I hope will soon become your Super Bod. In the next chapter we are going to concentrate on the most important, superficial, sign of ageing: the face and how to have Super Skin, naturally.

# 9.

# Super Skin

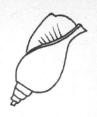

There are very few of us who don't want to look younger, and nowadays it's becoming nearly as 'normal' to have a quick nip and tuck as having your teeth whitened. Women as young as thirty-two are having regular Botox injections in their lunch hour and women as young as forty are having full facelifts. Cosmetic procedures have gone up by more than 300 per cent since the mid-1990s, and are likely to increase even more.

As the title of this book is *Alternative Ageing*, a full surgical facelift is not something I would consider. However, thanks to women like Sharon Osbourne and Anne Robinson, it is not something I can now say 'never' to! In the meantime, there are a lot of natural and not so natural options that can improve the appearance of the skin and, in some cases, look nearly as good as a facelift, without going near a knife. I will take you, briefly, through these semi-invasive options, talk you through the ones I've tried and finish with what you can do yourself, in the privacy of your own home. We've covered ageing from the inside out, now let's look at what we can do from the outside in.

But first, what causes all those lines people, usually relatives, refer to, kindly, as 'character' lines? Your skin is made up of damaged superficial cells and healthier deep cells. Every day your old superficial cells die, flake off and are replaced by younger cells. When you are born, this process only takes about a month. By the time you are sixty, it takes twice as long and the complexion becomes dull and lifeless because the cells on the skin's surface are, in fact, older.

By the time you are in your fifties, fine wrinkles and lines may have deepened into folds, especially around the mouth. Part of the reason is because, post-menopausally, there is much less oestrogen being produced, causing thinner skin. The skin is also less likely to retain moisture or produce collagen and elastin as efficiently. The result is baggy eyes, loose skin around the jaw, cheeks and chin and lots of 'character' lines around the mouth and eyes.

The muscles under the skin, like any other muscle in your body, lose their firmness unless they are exercised regularly. Thanks to gravity, the whole area starts heading south by middle age, and the lines deepen, especially if you spend your life scowling and frowning. So start smiling and make a decision now to do anything you can to help your face age gracefully before heading to the nearest plastic surgeon. First, let's start with the main skin agers and what we can do to avoid them.

## The Sun: Chief Skin Ager

There are dozens of reasons why our skin ages, but the predominant one is the reason we're all alive in the first place – the sun!

Sunbathing is responsible for 90 per cent of premature ageing of the skin, creating a large number of free radicals and damage to the collagen fibres that keep it strong and supple. (Just look at the skin on your buttocks to see how smooth skin looks that never sees sunlight!) Regular sunbathers can expect to add twenty years to their skin's age.

Some dermatologists think sunbeds have an even worse effect than direct sunlight because they give out even more damaging UVA rays, as well as increasing a risk of cataracts and skin cancer. A short high-pressure session on a sunbed can cause as much damage as a *year*'s normal exposure to the sun.

Professor John Hawk, consultant dermatologist at St Thomas' Hospital, London, fears an increase in skin cancers in the next few years as a result of regular use of sunbeds. He says that 'skin cancer can take twenty years to develop'.

SUN SENSE

- *Avoid strong sun, especially between the hours of 11 a.m. and 3 p.m. – even in the UK.*
- *Avoid the use of sunbeds.*
- *Don't get sunburnt.*
- *Wear a hat if you value your face.*
- *Use sunscreen, factor 15 and above.*
- *Get any moles that change shape or colour checked by your doctor.*
- *Be especially careful if you are very pale skinned and have freckles.*

## On the Other Hand

Sunlight is a key source of vitamin D and plays a crucial role in bone health and, more recently, has been discovered in research to regulate the production of cells, a mechanism that is absent in cancer. Professor Michael Holick, an endocrinologist from Boston University School of Medicine, believes his research could explain why people living in colder, northern climates, who get less vitamin D from the sun, have a higher risk of dying from colon, breast and prostate cancers. In Boston, he estimated that up to half of adults over fifty are vitamin-D deficient.

While he is not advocating sunburn, Professor Holick suggests that Caucasians spend five to ten minutes in the sun, unprotected, two to three times a week, applying protective creams if staying out any longer. Darker skins need a little longer in the sun to get the necessary amount of vitamin D from the UVB rays.

For completely different reasons, I totally agree with the professor and always spend up to fifteen minutes a day in the sun, without protection, but only before 11 a.m. or after 3 p.m. in the summer. It is well documented that people who cover themselves up in clothing from head to foot, for religious reasons, are more likely to suffer from rickets as children and from brittle bones and osteoporosis in later life because of a lack of vitamin D, which is essential for the bones to absorb calcium.

Natural daylight is also essential to trigger the pineal gland, to help you sleep better, and to help you avoid SAD during the winter. Try and get fifteen minutes of sunlight a day, during the safe times.

## Sunscreen – Pros and Cons

There is some controversy about whether we should be slapping on the sunscreen or not. A couple of years ago, EU scientists urged sunscreen makers to remove a chemical called methyl dibromo glutaronitrile, connected with a rise in rashes and allergic reactions and used in leading brands, from their products. Research published in the *British Medical Journal* also found that people who use sunscreen are *more* prone to skin cancer because it gives them a false confidence to sunbathe for longer and at the most dangerous times of the day.

Some skin experts advocate sunscreen all the time, others think that an over-protected skin will sag more and be thinner than skin that gets a little gentle sunshine and some sort of stimulation every day.

The decision must remain with you but, personally, I think there are so many chemicals and preservatives in sunscreens that I use a natural one. (There are several that only contain natural ingredients and antioxidants, up to SPF15.)

 TOP TIP

> *If you fancy mixing up your own sunscreen use zinc oxide – which is a total block, and used by surfers in Australia. Mix a little with a cold-pressed, unrefined vitamin-E-rich oil such as walnut, argan or even extra virgin olive oil. It will protect you and condition your skin at the same time.*

## After Sun Care

Remember all these polyphenols and vitamin E in extra virgin olive oil? In 2000, Japanese scientists discovered that basting the skin with the finest olive oil after sunbathing may protect it against skin cancer. Scientists at Kobe University School of Medicine carried out tests on GM hairless mice and found that high-grade virgin olive oil smeared on the skin delayed the appearance of tumours and reduced their size. The *New Scientist* also reported that the tumours were smaller, less frequent and there was less DNA damage to skin cells. European women have been using olive oil to keep their skin young for centuries, now I've joined them and have been using it as an after sun care ever since I read the research findings.

There are many other contributing factors to ageing skin, so here's a brief reminder of what causes wrinkles and what doesn't.

## Other Skin Agers

**Smoking**: the thousands of toxic chemicals in cigarette smoke produce free radicals that damage the skin and produce wrinkles. Smoking narrows the arteries and starves the skin of oxygen-producing lines, while constantly puckering the lips to inhale produces even more.

**Lack of sleep**: decreases keratin and collagen production. Growth hormones are mainly secreted at night and one of their main functions is to repair the body's tissues and encourage the skin to grow and heal. This process doesn't kick in until you have been asleep for six hours and given eight hours the skin will really look better.

**Stress**: is a major ager. Just see how much younger you look after a holiday. There are plenty of stress-busting exercises coming up on page 187.

**Air pollution**: living in a city can add five years to your skin's age. The constant onslaught of toxic pollutants causes more free radicals to form. A pathologist working in New Zealand told me that she found no difference between the lungs of smokers and people who have lived in cities! The anti-ageing diet and regular exfoliating will certainly help. Joining me living by the sea may help even more!

**Crash or yo yo dieting**: losing weight rapidly removes fat from the face too quickly and also causes the skin to sag and stretch.

**Unhealthy diet**: reduces the supply of nutrients and antioxidants to the skin as does . . .

**Poor digestion**: which we have tackled earlier on pages 152 and 153.

**A lack of essential fatty acids**: all the clients I see who have been on diets excluding all essential fats look ten years older than their age. Essential fats plump up your cells, big time.

**Not drinking enough water**: the process of skin ageing is primarily due to a loss of fluid. Drinking more than the minimum 1.5 litres of water a day will re-hydrate the cells and plump the skin right up.

**Lack of regular exercise**: means no freshly oxygenated blood is getting to the skin with its valuable nutrients.

**A sluggish lymph and liver**: we addressed both of these on pages 155 and 158. If you follow the advice, the quality of your skin will improve.

**Shallow breathing**: reduces the intake of oxygen which carries nutrients to the skin.

**Central heating**: really ages my skin. Put bowls of water in front of each radiator to humidify the air.

**Coffee, alcohol and anything containing caffeine or sugar**: all dehydrate the cells and cause glycation, which some experts liken to 'tanning a hide'.

## Natural Facelifts

Treating ageing from the outside is now a massive business. Non-invasive, natural 'facelift' treatments are available everywhere. Every beauty salon, on every high street, offers treatments such as CACI (computer aided cosmetology instrument), Hydra-Guinot lift and Carita Pro-Lift, that promise 'lifting' without surgery. I've tried most of them! They are expensive, because you need at least six to eight weekly sessions to really see any lasting benefits. They start at £50 a pop, and then you need one a month for maintenance. But they are cheaper than a surgical facelift, and they work. They are relaxing, non-invasive, natural and a wonderful option if you want to look really good for a particular occasion.

Another natural option, is facial acupuncture, which combines massage and acupuncture. The needles are used to stimulate the flow of energy (chi) and blood flow to specific points of the face. Needles can be used along facial lines, along the border of particular muscles or on specific acupuncture points. The treatment involves acupuncture all over the face, followed by a gentle derma roll, a kind of tiny prickly rolling pin, rolled across your face to increase circulation, followed by a fantastic facial massage using rejuvenating oils. This increases the circulation, relaxes the facial muscles and increases the elasticity of the skin.

Again, a course of treatments is recommended for the facial lines to soften and decrease and for the face to take on a healthy glow. Facial acupuncture improves the overall health of the facial tissue and changes should be noticeable after two or three treatments. But six–ten are usually recommended, costing in the region of £45 each. I had six and really noticed the benefits after the last one.

Julia Hancock, who trained at the International College of Oriental Medicine (ICOM) and who is also a member of the British Acupuncture Council, performed the treatment. She thinks this kind of anti-ageing treatment will last, especially if you follow a healthy lifestyle and watch your diet, and try not to be stressed out or scowl all the time. Julia has devised a massage you can do yourself at home, which you will find a little later, under the DIY section, on page 180.

## Semi-Invasive Treatments

Women tend to take after their mothers when it comes to facial ageing. They either age badly on the upper part of their face – baggy and droopy eyes, deep crow's feet and patchwork lines all over the face – or age below the nose – turkey-gobbler necks, jowls and droopy flesh around the mouth – sadly, that's the way I'm heading!

For the first group, there are some easy, not so natural treatments such as lasers, chemical peels, fillers and Botox, which many women consider from their early thirties on. I haven't tried any of them, but thousands of men and women swear by any or all of these alternatives to plastic surgery.

Problems with the lower part of the face – smile lines, called dynamic wrinkles – can be improved with laser resurfacing, dermabrasion, chemical peels, Botox and fillers such as collagen. If you hate your dynamic wrinkles that much, a reputable doctor should be able to give you all the pros and cons.

Then there are the fine wrinkles found on the cheeks on very dry, thin skin. These are superficial and can be removed relatively easily through skin care (more of that later), micro peels and other simple treatments.

## Permanent Natural Facelifts

Skin-fold wrinkles are the ones that go from the corner of the nose, around the mouth and down to the chin. They are called nasolabial folds and are the ones that upset me most. They are the result of sagging cheeks and the only way to tighten them is by tightening the skin, usually through a facelift. However, apart from exercising the muscles that lie underneath the skin, which would take another book to describe fully, I have found a natural alternative to delay the knife which I can vouch for, provided you are under fifty, or, preferably, even younger. It didn't work quite as well as I hoped because I think my cells were too old!

This is completely natural, non-surgical, non-invasive and non-toxic. It is dubbed holistic anti-ageing and is called Isolagen. Of the women who have used Isolagen, 75 per cent have never done anything else before. Unlike synthetic, and potentially unsafe products, Isolagen uses a process that treats the cause of ageing skin rather than the results. From a small skin sample, taken from behind your ear, they grow large numbers of new, healthy cells (fibroblasts) in a laboratory that are, uniquely, your own cells. These cells are fed and treated and generally given a bit of a holiday and after a couple of months, they are injected back into wherever you want them to go. However, some are cryogenically stored so they remain the age at which they were taken. And there's the rub. My cells were fifty-five when they were taken!

Once they are injected into your skin, these new, healthy fibroblasts get to work producing collagen to revitalize the areas of your face that show unwanted signs of ageing. Your new cells work to restore your skin, 24/7, year after year, reducing the signs of ageing and skin damage. This creates newer, healthier skin, with optimum results after about six months. There are two sets of injections and by the second set your wrinkles should have improved by 70 per cent.

For women who age on the upper half of their face and can get their cells stored when they are still young, I think this is a fantastic anti-ageing treatment. However, my cells weren't young and I chose the lower area, where the folds need a lot more help than my fibroblasts could give. But I did have them injected into my chest lines (very bad and crêpey from years of not wearing a bra and sunbathing foolishly in my youth), which was very painful but terribly successful. Those lines have improved considerably and I am very impressed. It is safe, economical and natural and definitely worth considering, especially if you are nearer forty than sixty. Isolagen has successfully treated 1,200 patients to date and no abnormal scarring or other adverse effects have been reported. There are nearly a hundred clinics in the UK and the treatment costs in the region of £3,000.

## Topical Creams

There is a new kid in town, when it comes to anti-ageing, called cosmeceuticals. These are topically applied creams and potions for acne, skin problems and anti-ageing that can be bought over the counter. They are more powerful than a lot of the so-called anti-ageing creams on the market, and have had a huge amount of money invested in research on them. I would need another chapter to describe in detail which ones are effective, but there are some key ingredients you should look for when buying these, potentially, expensive, but highly effective, treatments.

### KEY INGREDIENTS IN COSMECEUTICALS

- *Alpha lipoic acid: an antioxidant and anti-inflammatory*
- *Vitamin C ester: a collagen booster*
- *Dimetylaminoethanol (DMAE): when used in double-blind studies carried out by Johnson & Johnson, for N.V. Perricone M.D. Cosmeceuticals®, the skin was firmer, the lines minimized and the face was lifted*
- *Vitamin E: for skin health and lines*
- *Phosphatidyl-E: helps support the health of the cells' membranes*
- *Olive oil polyphenols: for preventing free-radical damage*

The best of the bunch, that include all these (patented) ingredients, is, without doubt, N.V. Perricone M.D. Cosmeceuticals. I have seen the before and after photographs taken for the Johnson & Johnson trials and the results are very impressive. However, they are not cheap and I haven't been able to afford them for long enough to tell you they dramatically lifted my face but, for the short time I used them, everyone kept saying how well I looked. As with everything in life, you get what you pay for. I have found cheaper brands, such as ROC, that contain more or less the same ingredients, but they don't produce such a dramatic effect.

However, if you look at the 'patented' ingredients, they can all be found in natural foods and some of them can be used separately in their original form. So you could experiment, like I do, and see how your skin reacts to any or all of them at home, using food you have already stocked up with.

### Cosmeceutical Ingredients in their Original Form

**Alpha lipoic acid**: is found in high quantities in meat. I'm stumped on this one, as I don't fancy a lump of meat on my face! But any antioxidant-rich fruit, such as papaya, is worth a try instead. Flaxseed oil, because of its high omega-3 content, should also be considered as an alternative because of its anti-inflammatory properties.

**Vitamin C ester**: available in liquid form from health stores, or straight from vitamin-C-rich foods.

**DMAE**: found in oily fish. You could try eating more oily fish, such as salmon, as well as using the oil from the fish-oil capsules topically – could be a bit smelly though – or take one 1000mg capsule with each meal.

**Vitamin E**: available in liquid form from health stores or you could use one of the vitamin-E-rich oils recommended in the DIY section on page 176.

**Phosphatidyl-E**: found in lecithin, so is really easy to use at home. Lecithin is also rich in acetylcholine – regarded as a moisturizer for the entire body. It is found in eggs, caviar, fish oils and olive oil, as well as lecithin. Caviar keeps popping up in some of the most expensive skin treatments on the market, so there must be something in it.

There are lots more ideas on what you can take out of your anti-ageing food cupboards and use *on* your face rather than eating on page 174. But first, let's take a look at the natural facelift options you can carry out in the privacy of your own home.

## DIY at Home

As you know, facial muscles are no different to any other muscle in your body in that they need exercising to keep them firm and toned. There are dozens of books and DVDs on sale explaining how to do facial exercises that produce good results. I prefer the really lazy option and have found a machine that does it all for me, without having to move a muscle, or look silly sitting in a traffic jam. It is like a mini Slendertone machine with electrode pads that stimulate the facial muscles to work harder. So I can sit watching TV *and* exercise.

There is serious science behind this particular machine. According to the manufacturers, Cleo, at about nineteen years old the signals from the brain to the muscles begin to slow down and consequently muscle starts to lose its firmness and tone. The Cleo 11 facial unit re-educates muscle fibre to work at the *correct* speed. Medically, this treatment is known as trophic neuromuscular stimulation (TNS) and was discovered by a physiotherapist treating Bell's palsy. Diana Farragher and her team developed this technology to regenerate the damaged nerve endings that lead to the facial paralysis common in Bell's palsy. But she noticed that one of the unexpected and most pleasing results was that her patients looked younger and their muscle tone had improved after treatment.

Like any fitness regime, it is best to do this as regularly as you work out the rest of your muscles – three to four times a week. And that's the only problem – I don't always have time to sit with pads all over my face, twitching away for an hour. It's difficult to read, work or do anything much other than watch TV. It is completely painless, though, and gives the face a very thorough workout. If I use the machine every night for a week, there is a very obvious improvement to my appearance. So, like all exercise, three to four times a week would really help towards a more permanently toned and lifted appearance and it's natural and cheaper than a facelift. The Cleo 11 costs in the region of £350 and is available from the website address in Resources on page 234. The company also sell other machines and pads for every part of the body, including the pelvic-floor muscles!

## DIY *Skin Care*

Let's take a look at what else you can do at home, with some of the oils and other foods you have hopefully bought for the anti-ageing diet. By the end of this chapter, you will be armed with all sorts of natural, rejuvenating fruit acids, exfoliators, moisturizers, toners and face packs – straight from your fridge or cupboard.

## Fruit Acids

Alpha hydroxy acid (AHA) fruit acids loosen the stiffness between dead-skin cells, so they fall away, leaving your face lovely and smooth and soft. You will find fruit acids in many natural foods including:

> All citrus fruit juices
> Live yogurt
> Grape juice
> Strawberries
> Digestive enzymes

Dab your chosen 'food' all over your face and leave it for ten minutes before rinsing off. Avoid the eye area and be careful in the sun if you use fruit acids every day, as you will be more likely to burn. Using these natural fruit acids really brightens and smooths the skin and you should see a difference in no time. Be careful, though, as some of them, especially lemon juice, can sting. A gentle alternative is a digestive enzyme, one that contains papain and bromelain, for example, which are natural fruit enzymes. I mix 1–2 capsules with a little water and apply it all over my face daily. And boy, can I see a difference to my skin when I don't!

## Exfoliators

Exfoliators and scrubs remove the dead cells, which clog up the skin and prevent it from retaining moisture. Regular exfoliating helps increase new collagen production and leaves your skin feeling softer, smoother and looking bright, healthy and more evenly toned.

You can exfoliate your entire body at the same time as you do your face, concentrating on any lumpy bits on thighs or arms. For extra moisturizing, mix one of these foods with your favourite 'carrier' oil until you have a small bowl full of gritty gunge! Exfoliate once or twice a week with one of these foods.

## NATURAL EXFOLIATORS

- *Ground sesame seeds (in fact, any seeds)*
- *Oatmeal*
- *Unrefined sea or crystal salt*
- *Bee pollen*
- *Kelp powder*
- *Lecithin granules*

## Moisturizers

Some of the oils mentioned earlier can double up as skin moisturizers because they are so rich in omega-3 and vitamin E, as well as antioxidants. You can use them all over your entire body, not just your face. They feed your skin with just what it needs to plump it out and make it look young again. My top three are flaxseed, argan and grapeseed oil, but if you haven't had a chance to buy any of them, you can always use extra virgin olive oil as it is rich in antioxidants and vitamin E.

### Flaxseed Oil
Flaxseed is *the* natural moisturizer because it contains the highest amount of omega-3 essential fats, which are needed by every cell in the body for optimum youth and health. Omega-3 improves the skin's condition and helps it stay young, healthy and flexible. This is my favourite rejuvenating oil and the one that has had the best results for me.

### Argan Oil
You can buy this oil ready blended for use at home (see Resources page 234). It is rich in vitamin E for neutralizing free radicals, and high in saponins that can slow down skin ageing and reduce wrinkles by increasing nutrients and oxygenation in the skin cells.

### Grapeseed Oil
Grapeseed oil is non-greasy and odourless so may be preferred by people who don't like the smell of the other oils. It is mildly

astringent and helps tighten and tone the skin. It is also high in antioxidants and omega-6 as well as containing decent amounts of vitamin E and bioflavonoids that help protect you against and neutralize free radicals.

There are many other excellent oils you can buy, such as wheat-germ, jojoba and sweet almond. But I have concentrated on the top three that were already on your shopping list for feeding your *internal* youth.

You may also like to invest in one or two essential oils, if you don't have them already. Not only can you use them to add to any of the above oils, as an extra moisturizer, you can also use them to add to your bath water for a nice relaxing soak, and they smell heavenly.

## HOW TO USE OILS

- *Face: use it as a rich nourishing facial oil at night, or to protect your skin in cold weather.*
- *Body: for dry skin, apply all over the body thirty minutes before a bath or shower.*
- *Nails: mix with lemon juice and soak nails for fifteen minutes once a week to strengthen them.*

## ANTI-AGEING ESSENTIAL OILS

- *Rose Absolute: the top of the pops when it comes to regenerating and smoothing your skin. If you only buy one, make it this one.*
- *Benzoin: tightens loose skin.*
- *Myrrh: strong firming qualities for saggy skin.*
- *Frankincense: skin-cell regenerator.*
- *Lemon: stimulates new, fresh cells.*
- *Lavender: very few people don't have this one lurking about in a cupboard. Relaxing but also stimulating and regenerating.*

Any of these oils can be added to your favourite carrier oil for moisturizing and massage. The ratio is: 2 drops of each essential oil to 30ml of carrier oil.

Here are a few other extras you may want to add to your anti-ageing potions.

## EXTRA SKIN SAVERS

- *Rose water: a skin-cell regenerator and a lovely toner.*
- *Vitamin C: encourages your collagen to grow and is perfect for round the mouth and lips to plump everything out. Buy it in liquid form.*
- *Vitamin E: the most important anti-ageing vitamin for the skin. Buy it in pure liquid form, not mixed with soya oil.*
- *Spirulina powder: improves the elasticity of the skin. It is rich in vitamin E, selenium and zinc for free-radical protection, and the high content of chlorophyll and tyrosine takes oxygen into the skin's cells and slows down the ageing process.*

## Toners and Tighteners

No beauty regime is complete without a quick tone to tighten the skin. Here are some natural alternatives that you can either find in your cupboard, fridge or local health store or chemist.

## NATURAL TONERS AND TIGHTENERS

- *Witch hazel*
- *Rosewater*
- *Lemon juice*
- *Cucumber juice*
- *Runny honey: apply as a mask, leave for five minutes, rinse off*
- *Egg white: whisk up two egg whites, apply as a mask, leave for five minutes and rinse off*

## Face Packs and Boosters

Finally, you may want to make a natural face pack. Here are a few ideas to give your skin an extra boost before a big night out.

*Natural Face Packs*
Mash a fresh avocado and add 1–2 capsules of kelp or spirulina to the mix. Apply to your face, neck and hands, then lie in a nice warm bath. This mixture is high in antioxidants, minerals and vitamin E to help stimulate fresh, new skin cells.

Blend half a cup of flaxseed oil, 2 capsules of kelp powder or spirulina, a heaped teaspoon of lecithin granules and/or a heaped teaspoon of bee pollen, the juice of a freshly squeezed lemon and half a cup of rosewater. Store in the fridge and use as a face pack for a pre-party boost.

### QUICK FIXES

- *Mineral-rich kelp or spirulina, slightly moistened, will give your skin a healthy glow.*
- *Lie down with cucumber slices all over your face. Cucumber is packed full of silicon and sulphur for strong skin and is very rejuvenating.*
- *Put green tea teabags on your eyes – full of antioxidants. Put them in water, squeeze them out and leave in the fridge for a couple of hours. Pop a tea bag onto each eye to add sparkle to tired eyes.*
- *Pure lemon juice applied after a moisturizer will give your skin a tightening, brightening effect.*

## Daily Regime

Here is my daily regime. If you follow this plan, with your own choice of natural products, you will see a great improvement to your skin tone and appearance in just two to three weeks.

- *Apply a digestive enzyme to exfoliate, stimulate and tone. Leave for five to ten minutes. Rinse off.*
- *Apply a hot flannel to open up the pores.*
- *Splash the face with cold water or tone using rose water.*
- *Apply an EFA moisturizer all over face.*

Here is a blend of oils for a first-class moisturizer.

½ cup flaxseed oil
½ cup rosewater
30 drops Rose Absolute
30 drops vitamin E

## Daily Rejuvenation Massage

Here is a daily facial rejuvenation massage, put together for you by Julia Hancock, the facial acupuncturist. First mix your preferred oil with your favourite essential oil and store it in a dark, glass bottle or any other air-tight container.

This massage should only take five minutes. Pull your hair off your face using a head band. Warm the oil between your palms and make sure there is enough to smooth all over the skin from the neck up, covering the face and forehead.

**Effleurage:** using both hands, and with a light, stroking movement, begin at the neck and make sweeping movements upwards, making sure the palms are in contact with your skin. Keep repeating, upwards over the neck, face and forehead. This improves the nutrition of the skin and tissues. Repeat five times.

**Mouth massage:** place the index and middle finger of one hand *above* the upper lip and the same fingers of the other hand *below* the lower lip. Pressing firmly, move both sets of fingers simultaneously around the mouth in a sweeping arc, so that they are always on opposite sides of the mouth. Work towards the corners of the mouth and back again in an arc. This works on the circular muscle around the mouth, reducing lines and tension. Repeat ten times.

**Eye massage:** using the tips of the middle fingers, firmly sweep in a circle from the inner corner of each eye, up and over the eyelid and down and around under the eye back to the corner, so you are completing a circle around the eyes. This helps circulation around the eyes, helps decrease puffiness, lines and dry, tired eyes. Repeat ten times.

**Forehead**: using the tips of the middle fingers of each hand, place them between the eyebrows so they meet. Rub the fingers briskly on the skin creating friction. Work upwards, to the hairline and repeat the process from the centre to the sides of your forehead till you have covered the whole forehead. Concentrate on any tense or lined areas. This is good for reducing tension and lines between the eyes and across the forehead. Repeat three times.

**Forehead**: place the hands on the forehead with the fingertips facing each other. Using strong, slow, firm movements, move the fingers away from the centre of the forehead, creating a sweeping pressure outwards with the fingertips. Repeat ten times.

**Face**: using the index and middle fingertips, make circular movements at the temples. Start off with deep pressure, becoming lighter with smaller circles before you move on. Do the same movement around the jaw, in front of the ears, gradually moving down until you reach the chin. Finally, carry out the same technique around the nasolabial folds, the lines from the side of the nostrils down to the corner of the mouth. Repeat until you feel that all the muscles have relaxed, releasing any tension in those areas.

**Invigorator**: if you want to finish with a quick 'wake up', tap briskly in a gentle slapping motion from the neck upwards, all over the face using stiff fingers. This will also wake up your circulation and, if you have time for nothing else, will do as a quick skin boost.

Apply vitamin C right at the end, round mouth and eyes.

I hope you have a chance to try some of these potions at home and find the facial massage as invigorating as I do. It certainly seems to be perking my skin up and improving its condition. Now your face is regaining some of its tone, it's time to look at the rest of the body and improve its appearance with some good old-fashioned, anti-ageing exercise!

# 10.

# Super Fit

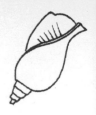

It was Hippocrates who said, 'to rest is to rust and to rust is to decay', and he's not wrong. Nothing will keep ageing at bay better than preventing that rusting. Most of us baby boomers are only too aware of how important exercise is to keep the joints, heart and skin young and healthy as well as keeping middle-age spread at bay. But most of us don't realize how much *more* we need to do to regain a toned, youthful body.

Research has shown that the basal metabolic rate (BMR) – the rate we burn calories when at rest – begins to decline from the age of thirty, along with the volume of lean muscle tissue. The result is an overall loss in lean body mass (LBM) and a gain in adipose tissue – fat! The sad fact is, that if we're not working our muscles as we age we are going to lose more than 3 kilos of muscle mass every decade, resulting in our metabolism slowing down by 2–5 per cent every ten years. That could mean an extra 6 kilos in weight by our mid-forties. Not only that, but the bones get weaker as the muscles get flabbier.

The good news is that by just putting on under 1.5 kilos of muscle mass you could increase your metabolism by as much as 7 per cent and turn yourself into a lean, mean, fighting machine. The bad news is, when you are over forty, and most definitely past fifty, you *cannot* lose weight effectively if you don't exercise at least four times a week. I am living proof of this.

Menopause expert Dr John Stevenson, from Endocrinology and Metabolic Medicine at the Faculty of Medicine, Imperial College, London, agrees that it's already difficult for women to maintain a healthy weight after the menopause because of hormonal and metabolic changes. 'Older women tend to carry body fat around the waist in an apple shape, much as men do,' says Dr Stevenson.

Weight carried in that area is linked to an increased risk of heart disease, and the sad truth is the older we are, the more we have to do to get rid of it. 'Post-menopausal women have to eat less or exercise more just to *maintain* their weight as they get older. But if you want to *lose* weight you need to eat less *and* increase activity,' Dr Stevenson says.

Don't worry, you don't need to hit the gym and start lifting dumb-bells three times a week to achieve this. People in the UK waste £200 million a year on unused gym memberships and there is no need to add to that figure! There are other ways to develop muscle mass without leaving home. I have integrated three different exercise regimes very easily into my busy life – and they're suitable for anyone at any age.

There are very many other reasons why exercise is anti-ageing, other than weight loss. Here are just a few to encourage you to increase your favourite exercise routine to at least four times a week:

## Reasons to Exercise

### Makes You Look Younger

Without exercise the lymphatic system doesn't work efficiently, so toxins and rubbish stay in the body and our lungs and heart work less, so our cells get less oxygenated, nutrient-rich blood. Every cell in your body is like a tiny factory. Better circulation and blood flow means more fuel and 'spare parts' arriving all the time for that little factory, so energy production stays high. As the circulation improves the lymph carries away waste and debris more efficiently. This results in cellular rejuvenation, which will make you look in blooming youthful good health!

### Stress

Twenty to forty minutes of aerobic exercise releases endorphins, those 'happy hormones' which are the body's natural painkillers, believed to be 200 times more powerful than morphine! Endorphin levels have been found to stay in the blood for as long as two hours after exercise, accounting for the well-known 'high' regular exercisers talk about. Stress symptoms such as depression and anger can disappear within twenty minutes of starting to exercise and regular sessions will help you have more energy, sleep better and have a clearer brain.

## Prevents Osteoporosis

Regular exercise helps maintain bone density, delaying the onset of osteoporosis. Women can lose up to 50 per cent of bone calcium by the age of ninety, increasing the risk of bone fractures. Physical exercise strengthens the bones and encourages the calcium to deposit in the right place. Weight-bearing exercise slows bone-density loss, improves balance and decreases the likelihood of slipping and breaking brittle bones. In studies done with women in their seventies, it was found that if they simply walked four times a week for twenty minutes, osteoporosis slowed down to almost pre-menopausal levels.

Anything that makes you go up and down on your joints has been found in scientific studies to be the best exercise to help prevent osteoporosis, with gentle jogging especially effective, but it doesn't suit everyone and brisk walking, especially uphill, is just as good.

## Prevents Heart Disease

Most people lose more than half their cardiovascular fitness between twenty and eighty. Exercise slows this loss right down. It also lowers blood pressure and cholesterol and cuts the risk of heart attacks by up to two thirds.

Regular aerobic exercise, as well as more gentle work-outs such as yoga, have been found to reduce the heart rate and blood pressure dramatically in only three months.

## Produces Growth Hormone

The secretion of one of the most important anti-ageing hormones, the growth hormone, declines between the ages of thirty and fifty causing muscles to shrink and fat to increase.

Fifteen minutes of exercise a day is enough to encourage the pituitary gland to produce more of this precious 'youth' hormone.

## Helps You Live Longer

A study carried out in America on more than 5,000 healthy centenarians found that some smoked, some drank alcohol, some ate red meat every day and some were non-smoking, non-drinking vegetarians. The one thing they had in common was that they worked up a good sweat every single day: jogging, chopping wood, making love, gardening or dancing. They all 'glowed' on a daily basis.

You may read this and decide you don't need to do anything else in the rest of the book to live a long and healthy life, and I wouldn't blame you! But how many of us do actually work up a sweat each and every day? Because of this simple top tip for longevity, I have included 'hot' yoga as one of my suggested exercises, but you could always have a daily sauna or steam instead although cardiovascular exercise has greater health benefits.

## Suppresses the Appetite

Finally, a half an hour or more of a light exercise such as brisk walking stimulates the secretion of epinephrine, which helps to suppress the appetite.

Before we get into what kind of exercise is best for you, there are a couple of checks to carry out. Just to cheer yourself up, here's a very simple test to see if you really are overweight. After that don't look at the scales again but go for maximum inch loss rather than maximum weight loss. A healthy weight range is based on a measurement known as the Body Mass Index (BMI), based on your height and weight.

---

*Ideal Weight Check*

Work out your height in metres and multiply the figure by itself.
Measure your weight in kilograms.
Divide the weight by the height squared (your first figure).

For example: if you are 1.6m (5 feet 3 inches) tall and weigh 65kg (10 stone) the figures stack up like this:

$1.6 \times 1.6 = 2.56.$
$65 \div 2.56 = 25.39.$

| | |
|---|---|
| BMI less than 18.5 | Underweight |
| BMI 18.5–25 | Ideal |
| BMI 25–30 | Overweight |
| BMI 30–40 | Should lose weight |
| BMI greater than 40 | It is essential to lose weight for the sake of your health. |

---

Hopefully, you have been pleasantly surprised and have discovered, as I did, that you are not overweight at all. You just have a little middle-aged spread to get rid of, and some toning to do.

If you find metric measures a bit of a pain, you can make life much easier for yourself by just going to any of the health websites and searching for BMI. I found a simple version on the BBC website. You will find the address at the back of the book (page 234).

Before you embark on any kind of exercise regime, however gentle, it might be an idea to check how fit you are. This is a very simple test you can do at home. You will need a step, stairs or something strong you can step onto that is 22 cm (9 in) high.

*Fitness Check*

Take your resting pulse. Finding your pulse, either on the side of your neck or on your wrist, count your pulse for ten seconds then multiply by six.
Step up and down the step or stair, using each leg, for a total of three minutes.
Stop. Rest for thirty seconds.
Take your pulse again.

*Result*
If your pulse goes up just a few beats above your resting pulse, you are at maximum fitness level.
If your pulse rate rises 10 beats above your resting pulse, you are at good to average fitness, with room for improvement.
If your pulse rate is more than 15 beats above your resting pulse, you need to start any exercise very slowly and build up gradually. If you have never exercised regularly before, or have been inactive for some time, have a health condition or are seriously overweight, please check with your doctor before embarking on any of the exercise suggestions.

## What Kind of Exercise?

For losing weight, firming muscle, toning and improving your heart, bone and joint health you need to do a combination of anaerobic and aerobic exercise. But I'm not talking about high-impact aerobic exercise such as running because it can be very stressful to the skeleton and can even displace organs as well as contribute to wrinkles. Aerobic means 'requiring oxygen' and how efficiently the body gets oxygen to the muscles. The stronger and healthier your heart, the more efficient your blood will be at doing this and the more aerobically fit you will become.

## AEROBIC EXERCISES

- *Brisk walking*
- *Dancing*
- *Yoga (hot, dynamic, Bikram or ashtanga)*
- *Cycling*
- *Swimming*
- *Keep-fit classes*
- *Treadmill*
- *Tennis*
- *Gentle jogging*
- *Rebounding*
- *Golf – as long as you walk fast between each hole!*
- *Gym machines – stair climbers or ski machines*
- *Skating or skiing*
- *Hill walking and rambling*

Anaerobic exercise requires less oxygen but does require muscular strength. Exercising your muscles, as in weight training, will burn fat fast. Remember, just putting on 1½ kilos of muscle mass will increase your metabolism by as much as 7 per cent and you will end up with a more chiselled and defined body.

## ANAEROBIC EXERCISES

- *Brisk walking while carrying weights*
- *Weight training*
- *Resistance training*
- *All yoga – you use your own limbs as weights*
- *Up- and downhill walking*

One of the best and easiest examples of combining aerobic and anaerobic exercise is power walking and carrying weights at the same time – uphill wherever possible. Wayne Leonard, an exercise physiologist, recommends 'interval training', which means two minutes of very fast walking, followed by one minute of slow walking. This gets the heart rate to rise rapidly then drop, which helps burn fat more effectively as well as exercising the heart.

## How Often, How Long?

To reduce body fat, you need to do a minimum of two to three sessions a week of weight or resistance training *plus* three sessions a week of aerobic exercise. Or, easier still, you can combine the two, as in hill walking with weights, for a minimum of four times a week.

Some research shows that doing short, repeated bouts of exercise actually burns more calories than doing one prolonged session. Others say you should be aiming for a minimum of fifteen minutes and a maximum of two hours' exercise a day. But it has to fit into your lifestyle or you won't do it. If it suits you better to do ten minutes in the morning, ten minutes at lunchtime and twenty minutes in the evening, that's better than doing nothing at all.

The exercises I think achieve the best all-round fitness for the older woman are yoga, walking and the Tibetan five rites which you can do at home. If you read my last book on weight loss, they will all be familiar to you. What won't be so familiar are the extraordinary anti-ageing benefits these exercises provide, as I have since discovered.

## Yoga

Yoga isn't just for super-fit celebrities who are so bendy they can get a foot behind their head. No matter how unfit, how old, how overweight or anti-exercise you are, you can practise yoga. It is just a matter of finding the right class.

Yoga is a 5,000-year-old ancient science, designed to unite body, mind and spirit. The postures and breathing exercises improve muscle strength and flexibility. It combines movement, relaxation, breathing and meditation. Regular practice will strengthen the body, increase flexibility and improve your mental focus and well-being. It also tones slack skin. One of the slimmest, fittest yogis I know is supple, healthy and vibrant without an ounce of loose skin or fat on her body. She's over seventy and has been practising daily since she was forty. She also goes on regular walking and hiking holidays.

Even the gentlest form of hatha yoga strengthens the whole body, tones the internal organs and stimulates the endocrine glands, which are so important for anti-ageing. Below are just a few of the long-term health benefits yoga will bring you if it is practised regularly:

### BENEFITS OF YOGA

Yoga alleviates:
- *Stress*
- *Insomnia*
- *PMS*
- *Asthma*
- *Arthritis*
- *Back pain*
- *Diabetes*
- *Constipation*
- *High blood pressure*
- *Headaches*

and improves
- *Circulation*
- *Digestion*
- *Muscle tone*
- *Cellulite*
- *Saggy skin*

If you want your yoga to be aerobic, muscle resistant and make you sweat, you need to look for a 'hot' yoga class such as Bikram, hot or dynamic yoga. The latter changed my life and my body shape in just three months of four sessions a week. I only lost a few kilos in weight, but I lost more than a few centimetres in flab as well as gaining sculpted shoulders, muscle definition and a slimmer tummy – and I dropped a full dress size!

Dynamic or hot yoga is based on powerful deep breathing and heat, and is inspired by many different kinds of yoga, including ashtanga. It is carried out in a heated room because, according to my teacher, Stuart Tranter, you are much less likely to injure yourself if you have a very warm body. 'The hotter you become, the more elastic your muscles, ligaments and tendons become,' says Stuart. It's a bit like metal that's hard and cold and extremely strong, but when heated becomes pliable and bendy. The heat also promotes sweating, 'which will flush toxins out of your body on a regular basis'.

As well as, hopefully, helping you reach the age of one hundred, this kind of yoga really works your heart. In a heated room, the heart rate goes up encouraging the body to use fat as a fuel almost immediately.

The minimum temperature recommended is 75 degrees, but anyone wanting to try Bikram yoga, be warned, the room is exceptionally hot at 110 degrees.

All types of yoga are muscle-resistant exercises because you use your own limbs as weights and counter weights, so you are carrying out weight training on your yoga mat with no other equipment but your body.

Whether you go for hot yoga or any other yoga, find a class that you get on with and where the room is well heated. Make sure it makes you sweat, breathe deeply and raises your heart rate. If it feels like twenty minutes, instead of the usual one and a half hours, you've found the right class.

## Walking – 10,000 Steps a Day

Well, you didn't think it would be just a stroll in the park did you? It may sound like an awful lot of walking, but 10,000 steps a day is far easier to accomplish than you might think. It amounts to about 4 miles. If you buy a pedometer – often given away in cereal packets – you will find you can soon build up to 10,000 steps, especially if you take smaller strides.

In the 1950s people were far more likely to accomplish 10,000 steps a day because they walked further as part of a daily routine. We used to walk to the shops and to school, play outside because there was little TV to watch, even if we owned one, and not every family owned a car.

Dr John Buckley of Keele University tested out a 10,000-steps-a-day plan on one of Britain's laziest groups of this century – students – to see if what he calls a 'small amount of exercise' would improve their health. Over four weeks the students, who previously had never done any exercise, walked the required number of steps a day. The results showed that their stamina improved, they felt fitter and their hearts and lungs improved by 3 per cent in just a month.

According to Dr Buckley, over a lifetime all those extra steps could reduce the risk of obesity, heart disease and stroke. And if that doesn't convince you, hopefully this will.

If you were to walk briskly for forty-five minutes a day, four times a week, you would lose 8 kilos in a year. Without dieting. Apart from strengthening your heart and lungs, walking works all the lower-body muscles, improves bone density and puts less stress on the joints than running or jogging. Walking is the most frequently prescribed form of exercise when it comes to preventing conditions such as osteoarthritis and osteoporosis, as well as chronic backache, which plagues 10 million of us a year, in the UK alone.

Studies of walkers who walk in excess of 5 mph (that's very fast) estimate they burn *twice* as many calories as runners travelling at the same pace, because they use more muscle groups. It is also a more 'resistant' type of exercise than jogging because you tend to use your arms more and take longer strides.

Finally, you can walk anywhere, anytime and don't need any special clothes or equipment to start, unless you want to add some hand weights and special toning shoes.

TWENTY TOP TIPS FOR BUILDING UP TO 10,000 STEPS A DAY

1. *Take smaller steps than normal. Fast, short steps will work you harder and get you to 10,000 quicker.*
2. *Build up slowly, starting off with 1,000 steps or ten minutes a day.*
3. *Don't try and accomplish 10,000 steps in one go, break it into sections.*
4. *Make sure your head and shoulders are relaxed.*
5. *Walk to the local shops instead of using the car and use a shopping trolley or rucksack to carry your shopping home.*
6. *Get off the bus or train one stop earlier and walk.*
7. *Go out for a walk at lunchtime.*
8. *Walk the children, or grandchildren, to and from school.*
9. *If you play golf, walk as fast as possible between holes.*
10. *Park your car in the furthest bay away from the supermarket doors.*
11. *Aim to walk as if you have a bus to catch rather than dawdling along.*
12. *Walk fast enough to gently 'glow', but slow enough to carry on a conversation.*
13. *Even if you live in a city, find a hilly area and walk uphill to work your heart harder.*
14. *Walking downhill also increases aerobic activity because you are using different muscles as shock absorbers.*
15. *Take a Pac a Mac instead of an umbrella.*
16. *Wear loose comfortable clothes and good trainers.*
17. *Pump your arms to work your heart more.*
18. *Hold a small bottle of water in each hand to use as weights.*
19. *At the end of your walk, slow down and cool down.*
20. *Stretch all the muscles you've been using.*

If you really want an extra workout while you are out walking, I have found a trainer called a multi-gym in a shoe! I discovered Masai Barefoot Technology (MBT) a couple of years ago and found the shoes so beneficial I became an MBT trainer and regularly run power-walking classes for the ladies of Brighton.

MBTs have become very well known in the UK press for their ability to reduce cellulite and tone muscle better than any other shoe. However, they were actually designed by scientists in Switzerland as a rehabilitating, orthopaedic shoe to help people realign their skeletal structure and improve any problems with gait, knees, hips and feet. They do this by making you walk as you would if you were barefoot on the sand, making you walk straighter, reducing the load on your spine and joints and relieving tension. The shoes make you roll instead of repeating the shocks and compressions that other trainers do, and are particularly suitable for the over fifties. Here are just a few things MBTs may help:

> Muscle tone
> Reduce cellulite
> Varicose veins
> Reduce weight
> Improve circulation
> Improve posture and balance

Walking in MBTs helps strengthen the ankles, knees, hips and spinal joints. Blood circulation is increased and the whole body lengthens and strengthens. Because you are walking as upright as a Masai, your joints are aligned correctly allowing your tendons and muscles to support you instead of overloading and stressing your joints. This is particularly important for anyone with osteoarthritis, osteoporosis or any other degenerative diseases of the bones and joints.

Most muscular and skeletal problems originate from poor posture and faulty gait patterns. MBTs change your stance so you walk in a straight, elegant, balanced and comfortable manner, which is kind to your joints, while gently stabilizing your pelvis and spine. You walk like a model! Because of the therapeutic benefits these shoes are classed as medical equipment in the EU.

As important, according to Lisa Dann, fitness consultant, you burn up to three times as many calories when you walk in these shoes, so they help you to lose weight. She says her mother uses them when she plays golf and has toned her muscles and lost weight.

Add hand weights, and you really do have a gym in a shoe. I use these shoes for a workout in between yoga and try and do my 10,000 steps a day when I'm wearing them. They're not the cheapest or most attractive shoes in the world but, as trainers, they do far more than any other. Don't forget to take smaller steps than normal. It's very important for your gait and you will get to 10,000 much quicker. I recommend to clients that they walk to work in them, or part of the way, change when they get to the office, and wear them again to walk home. If you use these shoes with weights and do 10,000 steps you don't need to do much else.

## Tibetan Five Rites

You may have come across these exercises in the *Weekend Weight Loss Plan*. What I didn't know then is how good they are for longevity as well. So here they are again.

Fellow nutritionist Nor Power taught me the Tibetan five rites. Nor discovered these five simple exercises ten years ago having come across them in a book. She used to do 50–100 sit-ups for her abs and other toning exercises for the rest of her body. But, having given the five rites a whirl, she noticed, even after the very first day, that her muscles ached more than they had after her other regime. She had better ab definition doing just twenty-one of each of the five rites than with her previous hundred sit-ups. She felt more energetic and noticed that these simple exercises gave her back, tummy, thighs, arms and shoulders a thorough, but quick, workout.

These simple exercises will wake up your whole endocrine system and, as you are working your whole body using your own limbs as weights, will also tone and strengthen the major muscle groups, serving as quick muscle-resistant exercises you can do at home. More importantly they are anti-ageing.

## Why the Five Rites Reverse Ageing

The Tibetan monks, who originated these exercises many hundreds of years ago, believe that an energy centre or vortex covers each of the major seven endocrine glands. Hindus and yogis call them chakras. In a healthy body, each vortex revolves at great speed allowing life energy, or prana, to flow upward through the endocrine system. If one of them slows down, the flow of health and vitality gets blocked and that particular gland may not work as efficiently as it should.

The quickest way to regain youth, health and vitality is to start these energy centres spinning normally so that each of the vortexes revolves at great speed, permitting vital life energy to flow upward through the endocrine system.

When they are all revolving at the same speed your nerves, organs and glands will work better and you will age better.

Bruce Forsyth still tap dances in his seventies and I have seen him do the first of these exercises on TV and credit them for his health and vitality. Whether you choose to believe that they can postpone ageing and restore a youthful appearance or not, many followers, including me, do report having a calmer and clearer mind and feel much better for doing them because they help circulate oxygen to the brain. Whether they stimulate the chakras, or energy centres, or the endocrine system, they certainly energize me and I feel much less centred and more sluggish when I *haven't* done them.

Either way, they give your body a very good and quick workout, using all your main muscle groups.

## How to Do the Five Rites

For the best results these rites need to be done daily. They will only take ten minutes to do, once you've learnt them, and within a month of daily practice you should look and feel more vibrant.

Each exercise should be repeated no more than twenty-one times. But most of us need to work up to that number. So start with as many as feels comfortable and increase the number each week. If you can only manage three repetitions at first, that's fine. Increase it to five or six the following week, and so on.

Everyone is different; so if you get stuck on nine repetitions and can't seem to get past that number, don't push yourself. Listen to your body and do what you're comfortable with. It doesn't matter *when* you get to the point of being able to do twenty-one repetitions, as long as you're doing them daily. Eventually you'll be doing them all in just ten minutes before rushing off to work or out for the day.

## Exercise One

This exercise will also be familiar to you if you have read my book *48 Hours to a Healthier Life*. It might make you feel like a mad whirling Dervish or a child, but it will help wake everything up and is a great stress-buster. If you do nothing else, do this one. The Hale Clinic's ayurvedic doctor, Doja Purkit, recommends that we all spin if we want a stress-free day. 'If you can spin twenty times you will never feel stress', he says. Dr Purkit believes spinning replicates the turbulence caused by stress in the body's cells and helps the body to understand and overcome it.

Stand up straight with your arms stretched out to the sides. Palms open and facing downward. Spin round clockwise until you become dizzy – usually five or six times, the first time. Make sure your feet are squarely on the ground throughout, and spin as fast as you can without falling over. Stand still at the end and take a couple of full, deep breaths.

To help combat dizziness, you could try the trick that dancers and skaters use. Fix your eyes on an object or a mark on the wall in front of you, level with your eyes, and keep your eyes on that point for as long as possible while you are turning. Your head will have to keep up with your body, but turn your head at the last possible moment really quickly so you can stare at the same spot as you come round. Be careful not to hurt your neck by moving it too quickly.

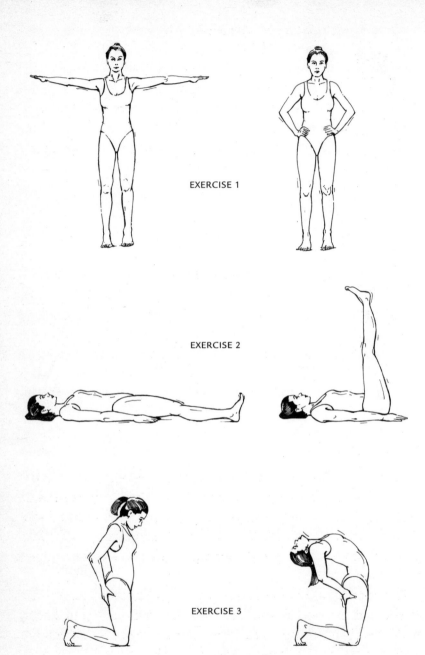

EXERCISE 1

EXERCISE 2

EXERCISE 3

EXERCISE 4

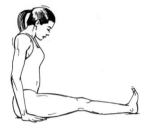
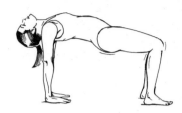

EXERCISE 5

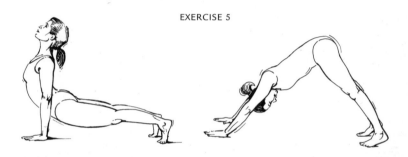

## Exercise Two

Lie flat on the floor, preferably on a thick carpet or rug, face up. Put your arms down by your sides, palms facing down. Inhale deeply and lift both your legs vertically just past a 90-degree angle. Raise your head off the floor with your chin tucked in. Your toes point towards the ceiling and your lower back should remain glued to the floor.

Exhale and lower both your head and legs. Repeat as many times as you can manage. If you can't initially straighten your knees, keep them bent till you can. The important thing is that you are working your abs and thighs, not your neck.

Take two full breaths before moving on to the next exercise.

### Exercise Three

Kneel on the floor, upright, with your hands on the back of your thighs or just below your bottom. Your knees should be about 10 cm (4 in) apart. Look down, tucking your chin in, then inhale and drop your head as far back as you comfortably can arching your back from the waist. Use your arms and hands for support as you lean back. Exhale as you return to the starting position and repeat as many times as you can.

Take two deep breaths before moving on to the next exercise.

### Exercise Four

Sit on the floor with your legs straight out in front of you with your feet about 30 cm (12 in) apart and your back straight. Your palms should be face down on the floor parallel with your hips. Tuck your chin into your chest. Inhale through the nose, and raise your hips as you bend your knees, pushing your whole body up, like a crab. Then drop your head back as far as it will go and, at the same time, tense your muscles. Your arms should be straight and your feet shouldn't move as you exhale and come down to the starting position.

Take two deep breaths and turn onto your tummy.

### Exercise Five

The last exercise is the one I find the toughest. It really works the arms, thighs and abs. Lying face down on the floor have your legs hip-width apart, toes tucked under. Your hands are palm down next to your ears. Lift yourself off the floor, as if you are hovering, by supporting yourself on the palms of your hands and the balls of your feet. Your head is up and back.

Inhale and push yourself up into an inverted V, so your arms and legs are straight, by raising your bottom and tucking your chin into your chest. Exhale as you lower yourself back down keeping your body off the ground in that hovering position.

Stand up and take two deep breaths, then lie down and relax for a couple of minutes until your breath returns to normal.

That's it, five simple exercises that have given your muscles and glands a quick but thorough workout.

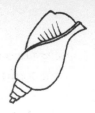

## 11.

# Super Life

We have looked at what you need to put into your body, on your body and how to look after it from the outside in and the inside out. This is the chapter that will hopefully empower and inspire you in all other areas of your life. So far, we haven't had a real look at the emotional and spiritual side of our lives and how the biggest cause of ill health and ageing can be avoided with a few simple techniques to help still the mind and the spirit, as well as the body.

## Super Stress Busters

You have already read what stress does to us at a cellular level. This section is going to help you learn how to cope with stress *from* a cellular level. One of the few hormones that increase with age is the stress hormone, cortisol. In excessive amounts it can kill brain cells and weaken the immune system as well as decreasing muscle mass and ageing the skin. It is known as the 'death hormone' in the anti-ageing field for a very good reason. Excessive and prolonged production of cortisol seems to be the biggest underlying cause behind almost every illness, from cancer and heart disease to constant colds and skin conditions.

### The Four Stages of Stress

**People poisoning**: emotionally draining friends, a bullying boss, an unhappy partner or a stroppy client. People can make you feel constantly angry and worthless. Give them up! The biggest drains on your emotional bank are emotional vampires: the friends or family who talk about themselves incessantly and rarely listen to you; the ones who moan constantly. Restrict the time you spend with negative friends and family, especially the ones who constantly repeat negative statements like 'All men are bastards,' 'You're too long in the tooth for that,' etc., etc.

**Doing too much**: in the UK we have the longest working hours in Europe, and have all turned into hamsters going round and round and round on a treadmill without stopping for breath. No one is going to put, 'I wish I'd spent more time working' on their gravestone! Pace yourself and learn to relax. Our cells need to rest to regenerate. Getting rid of tension in the body by relaxing for as little as ten to twenty minutes a day, can be almost as good as a night's sleep for cell regeneration.

**Sleep deprivation**: we looked at the causes of insomnia earlier in the book, but the relaxation techniques and exercises coming up on pages 207–9 will really help you sleep better at night. If you *have* been up all night, a fifteen-minute nap (no more) will help – so grab a quick quarter of an hour when you can.

**Life-changing events too close together**: the death of a spouse or a loved one, severe illness, a major operation, divorce, being made redundant or retiring are all common occurrences by the time we get to middle age. Try not to make any big decisions in your life for a year after such a crisis. For example, don't move house straight after bereavement. A mind-mapping exercise described on page 221 will help you make major decisions, as will all the stress-busting techniques coming up.

Most of us in the West have enough to eat and a roof over our heads, but we live in a constant state of mental and emotional stress. We worry about our relationships, work and money. We worry about our families, crime, the terrorist threat and our environment. We probably worry more now than ever before! We need to stop worrying about things that are beyond our control. The only way to do that is to find more time to look after yourself, instead of worrying about everyone else.

Remember that prolonged stress results in a run down immune system, which can lead to disease and an ageing face and body.

Here are some suggestions on how to de-stress and feel happier about yourself on a daily basis.

The first step is to turn all negatives into positives! Remember that list of emotional agers way back in Super Agers on page 9: unhealthy relationship, stressful job, stressful home life, little or no exercise, little or no fresh air or sunlight, always on the go, don't meditate, don't do breathing exercises, don't do yoga or tai chi, no time to just sit and be, no time to relax, no time for me? They must now become positive anti-ageing goals.

## Positive Attitude

Optimists generally live longer, happier and healthier lives. Studies constantly prove that we can feel better about anything if we have a positive attitude towards it, so we need to change any negative thoughts into positive ones from now on; change every thought about the past or the future into the present. And really *think* it. If you constantly say something in the future tense, I want to be . . . I wish for . . . it will stay in the future. That's how obedient the subconscious mind is. But say it in the present and it becomes the now. Instead of thinking: 'I will never find a car parking space' start thinking, 'There's a space for me now.' It really works!

I know it all sounds a bit weird, but if you trust that the universe or your god will provide you with whatever you need, including a long and youthful life, it does. But never forget to say thank you!

Say this positive affirmation in front of the mirror. 'I am ageing remarkably well, and looking vibrant, healthy and fit.' If you say it enough times your subconscious will take it as read and your cells will deliver. Did I say will? I mean, they *are* delivering as we speak!

## Time for Exercise

We've discussed how important exercise is for busting stress and keeping you young and healthy. Thirty minutes, five days a week is only one and a half hours of your total week. Now tell me you don't have time. Get into the habit of at least half an hour, preferably 10,000 steps (page 191), every single day to sweat stress and toxins out of your body. If you can't find time, do the gardening, make love or dance around the kitchen listening to loud music. It doesn't matter, as long as you move enough to release those happy endorphin hormones. Anything that oxygenates the blood makes controlling stress much easier.

## Time for Fresh Air and Sunlight

Getting outside as often as you can feeds the pineal gland with light so you sleep better. Melatonin, the chemical produced by the pineal in response to light, is the only chemical that affects every single cell in the body.

Dr Stephany Biello of the Department of Psychology at the University of Glasgow, who is researching into biological timing and sleep, says that, 'For many older individuals, light later on in the day and early evening has been shown to be the most beneficial', probably because we have slightly earlier circadian phases than younger adults. 'A combination of bright light and exercise helps improve how older people function during the day, because it increases slow-wave sleep which, in turn, helps daytime performance.'

## Time to Meditate

Meditation helps us slow down, inside and out. It may even slow the ageing process. Those practising for five years or more appear, on average, five years younger than their actual age. Meditators use doctors almost half as much, heart disease is 80 per cent lower and cancer is 50 per cent lower. Dr Jay Glaser, a research physician, discovered why people who meditate regularly seem younger than their chronological age: their levels of the anti-ageing hormone DHEA were significantly higher. Meditating people over forty-five have up to 47 per cent more DHEA, completely independent of diet, exercise, weight and alcohol consumption.

Improved DHEA levels reduce body fat, improve skin texture, moisture and tone, increase sex drive and improve immunity, memory and bone density. It keeps weight down, and helps people look younger.

You don't need to sit cross-legged on the floor for two hours a day. Even if it's only five minutes a day, meditating regularly will reduce stress and fatigue and keep you young. If you think you don't have time, more words of wisdom from Mahatma Gandhi, who apparently said, 'I have so much to do today I will need to meditate twice as long.' You will find a good meditation practice on page 228.

## TOP TIP

*Believe it or not, just sitting cross-legged under a tree, making sure your back is in touch with the trunk, can have the most de-stressing effect. If you don't have time for the breathing or meditation exercises on the next few pages, try this instead for just five minutes and see how grounded and calm you feel. People always make fun of hippies who hug trees, but I think there's something in it. If you believe, as I do, that every 'life' on this planet is linked in some way then the life force and energy that is contained in a two-hundred-year-old tree must have some effect on us at a cellular level. Try it – you've nothing to lose though you may get strange looks from passers by.*

## Time to Breathe

Pranayama is yogic breathing. It increases your intake of that precious vitamin O – oxygen – to give you life, energy and a sharp brain. Pranayama recharges your batteries and calms down your mental state by regulating the flow of prana or chi, known in Eastern practices as vital energy believed to circulate round the body in currents. But the most important reason to do pranayama, I believe, is because of its effect on your brain. We know that there are two hemispheres in the brain with different functions: the left for logic, languages and figures; the right for creativity, imagination and intuition. By inhaling through alternate nostrils you send the breath to each side of the brain in turn which will help balance the two hemispheres. This is known as a neuromuscular integration, which basically means you are integrating mind and body and creating greater mental clarity and energy.

If you don't fancy meditating or hugging a tree, pranayama is a
really easy exercise to do anywhere – in the car, on the train, or,
preferably, outside in a park or, as I do, by some oxygenating water.

## PRANAYAMA BENEFITS

- *Expels stress*
- *Increases oxygen*
- *Improves digestion*
- *Stills the mind*
- *Recharges the batteries*
- *Increases physical energy*
- *Increases mental clarity*
- *Relaxes you*
- *Works as a quick meditation*

*Pranayama*

Sit comfortably facing the sun, with your spine as straight as
possible. Close your eyes and rest your left hand on your left knee.
Using your right thumb, close your right nostril. Then inhale
slowly and deeply through your left nostril. Hold the breath for
four counts. Using your two middle fingers of the right hand, close
your left nostril and slowly exhale through your right nostril. Keep
your left nostril closed and inhale through your right nostril. Hold
the breath for four counts. Move your thumb onto your right
nostril and exhale through the left nostril. Repeat the sequence for
about five minutes.

Your breathing may be slightly slower and deeper than usual,
but it should be natural and unforced. When you are finished, sit
quietly for a few minutes and breathe normally.

## Time For Yoga or Tai Chi

Exercise like yoga or tai chi has been found to reduce the heart
rate and blood pressure dramatically in just three months. Stress
symptoms such as anxiety, depression and anger can disappear
within twenty minutes on the very first day. Most regular devotees

of these gentle Eastern practices report having more energy, sleeping better and experiencing a clearer mind. They help you change your negative thoughts and energies into positive thoughts and energies. They help balance ying and yang for perfect harmony.

You already know about the benefits of yoga, but in case you don't know about tai chi – the exercise that Chinese workers do in the park every single morning before work – here's a quick description. Tai chi chuan, incorporating chi kung, has been around for more than 10,000 years. It is a series of moves put together to create harmony for the mind, body and spirit. It is a moving meditation, a powerful tool for relaxation as well as self-defence. It can increase focus, concentration and clarity of mind and regular practice allows the chi, or energy, to flow and circulate throughout the whole body, improving your posture, self-esteem and metabolic rate. Most importantly, tai chi really helps the adrenals: the glands that produce all that stress in the first place!

Learning tai chi is one of my new things this year, so you may see me on the beach gliding through the movements, gracefully, I hope! If you fancy learning too, there is a website where you can find out more listed in Resources on page 234.

## Time to Sit and Be

### Muscle Relaxation

Try this very simple relaxation exercise whenever you are stressed. The body is stilled by complete relaxation. It eases tension in the muscles and rests the whole system leaving you as refreshed as after a good night's sleep. It carries over into all your activities and teaches you to conserve your energy and let go of worries and fears. It also serves as a great pick me up if you are going out straight after work and feel exhausted. It helps you relax in bed at night if you are having trouble sleeping. This position is also fantastic for easing backache and is something my body just loves after hours at the computer.

Sit on the floor, on the carpet or a thick towel, with your bottom resting on your heels. With the spine straight, lift your arms over your head and put your hands together in a 'prayer' position. Your fingers point up to the ceiling. Stretch the arms up and then drop them down onto the floor stretched out in front of you. Your forehead should be on the ground, and your bottom as close to your heels as you can manage. Relax and let everything go. Stay like that for a full five minutes. Roll up gently to return to the original position, stretching your arms once more above your head, with hands in prayer position, for one last stretch. Get up slowly. You should feel thoroughly relaxed and the discs in your spine will be nice and plumped up.

## Time to Relax

There are lots of other ways to relax, but one of the best by far, I'm sure you'll agree, is having a long hot soak in the bath. Warm baths open the pores and create sweating, and help to open the cells and release toxins. They also lower blood-sugar levels, relieve painful joints and muscles and improve colon peristalsis (moving your bowels).

My favourite bath is an Epsom salt bath because of the effect it has on the cells. Remember that magnesium, potassium lesson on page 51? Epsom salts are actually made of magnesium sulphate. This is one of the minerals we want to get back *into* the cells to help us detoxify and improve the electrolyte balance. Magnesium also relaxes the muscles, big time. Soaking in Epsom salts will *increase sweating* and help any muscular aches and pains you might have. It is also very good for people suffering from arthritis or sciatica and will help fight colds, flu and other viruses.

Any sea salt or essential oil will also help you relax at bath time and sleep like the dead, but if you want to have an Epsom salt bath, follow the instructions on page 230. Always drink plenty of extra water before, during and after your bath because the heat and sweating will dehydrate you.

## Time for Me

The week I gave up watching TV, I got so much done that I wondered why I hadn't done this for more than a couple of days ever before. If you want more time for yourself, this is the thing to do. I recently read an inspiring article about the Barefoot Doctor and how he, an ex-hippy, runs a collective in Spain, has written a dozen books, made a CD called *Om*, has a TV series, makes a range of health drinks, markets smellies *and* remains calm and un-stressed. How does he fit it all in? I feel exhausted just writing that list of accomplishments. He was quoted as saying, 'I don't watch telly. I get these ideas and then I have to do them.'

While watching TV you are exposed to frequencies that vibrate twenty times faster than our brain waves, which results in a lack of concentration, nervousness and insomnia. And the body produces additional free radicals. Cut down your viewing and spend more time doing those 10,000 steps.

There are many other things you can do to give yourself time for you, but the most beneficial has to be massage. It will make you feel loved, nurtured, relaxed and happy.

### Massage

Book yourself in for a regular massage. You don't have to spend a lot of money as there are always local colleges needing 'guinea pigs', or you can give yourself one at home. There's one on page 231 you might like.

The best type of massage, for de-stressing and anti-ageing, is an aromatherapy massage. Essential oils are used to massage your muscles and help your blood and lymph flow better. You can choose oils that will help balance your hormones, help you sleep or re-energize you. Oils pass through the skin into the bloodstream and can influence your entire body's health as well as your mental wellbeing.

## Super Happiness

Nothing makes you look younger or relieves tension quite like laughing. Having a good laugh melts away stress, lowers blood pressure and oxygenates the blood. All that lovely nutrient-rich blood is encouraged to go straight to your face to give you a youthful bloom. All those happy hormones also strengthen your immune system. Recent research has shown that healthy people are usually happy people. When you smile, your body manufactures different chemicals than those it produces when you feel bitter and twisted. Watch comedies instead of the news, hire funny films instead of violent ones, and laugh yourself healthy and young.

When you smile, imagine you are smiling through your whole body. It really will make a difference to the way people react towards you. I know this sounds very hippy dippy, but when you give out love that's exactly what you get back. Recently, I took an instant dislike to someone in the same singing class as me. I found her rude and obnoxious. One day I was standing behind her thinking how horrible she was, when I remembered what I am advising now! I put out loving thoughts, saying to myself that maybe she was rude and sarcastic because she was overweight and suffered from low self-esteem. Do you know, the most amazing thing happened, five minutes later she turned round and complemented me on something I was wearing. We've been friends ever since. Try it next time you are thinking grumpy thoughts. It really works.

### Do Things that Bring You Joy

Act your shoe size! Be childlike and learn how to feel completely unselfconscious. Do something silly, like launching yourself down a slide in a children's playground. Remember, short bursts of adrenaline produce more natural killer cells. So what are you waiting for? Take up roller-blading, jump out of a plane, climb a mountain. You are never too old, provided you are fit. There's a club in Brighton for people between thirty and sixty-nine who love dancing. If the baby boomers are anything to go by, I don't think it will be too long before there are raves for sixty- to eighty-year-olds, and I will be first in line!

If you only had one week left to live, what is it you have never done and have always wanted to do? The statement 'life isn't a dress rehearsal' couldn't be truer, what are we all waiting for?

## Travel

I backpacked, on my own, around Thailand at the age of fifty and last year went round the world, aged fifty-five. But I'm not that unusual. There's a whole new breed of baby boomers who have two things in common: age is not going to stop them doing anything they want and they are spending the kids' inheritance now! Only this weekend, I heard of a sixty-year-old woman who had spent a year learning different dances in different countries round the world, because that was her passion. She learned to salsa in Cuba, tango in Buenos Aires and hula in the Cook Islands.

She isn't alone, according to Lonely Planet's Laetitia Clapton. Gap years are no longer for the young. More and more baby boomers are turning to the delights of adventurous and unplanned travel. It is not unusual for Laetitia to come across a seventy-four-year-old who wants to climb Mount Kilimanjaro or motorcycle across America.

## Education

A friend of mine has just given up her job at the age of forty and is doing a two-year MA degree. If you didn't have the chance to go to university, now's your chance, it is *never* too late. My step-father won a scholarship to Oxford when he was eighteen but got waylaid by the war, marriage, children and a career. He finally got round to doing a history degree at sixty-five. He did tell me he kept forgetting he had already attended certain lectures, but he still gained a respectable 2.1.

Learning something new exercises your brain and keeps you

young. Take an art class, learn a foreign language, go for dancing lessons. It doesn't matter what it is. Stimulation is associated with a decreased risk of Alzheimer's and other brain-ageing conditions. You may have the leisure and the money for the first time in your life to try things you have always wanted to do. Read how to use the mind-mapping exercise on page 221 to see what missed opportunity you could take up.

## TOP TIP

*If you want more time and energy here is a top tip from life coach, Conor Patterson. When you wake up, get up immediately, what- ever the time, as long as the sun has risen. (It is much easier to do this in the winter!) Try it for two weeks, it will take your body that long to adjust, but you will find you have a lot more energy and time. When you wake up and look at your watch and think, 'It's only 6.30 in the morning what on earth do I need to get up now for?' don't listen to yourself. Conor says the body is awake for the good reason that it has had enough rest. And it works. Many of you reading this already get up at the crack of dawn but, until I discovered this technique, I wasn't one of them.*

## Sex

Put the passion back into your life! People who have frequent sex live longer than those who don't. Sex lowers cholesterol levels, boosts blood circulation and releases endorphins. There is even evidence that frequent ejaculations reduce men's risk of prostate cancer by a third. Have sex with your partner or on your own, it keeps you looking young.

If you don't have a partner or lover and want one, make it a goal. No one meets anyone staying at home and refusing to go out. Sadly, prospective partners don't come and knock on the door. Join a dating agency, answer a personal ad or put one in yourself, making sure of the usual safety precautions. And yes, I'm going to say all the usual stuff about joining groups: dancing, singing, theatre, poetry, rambling, bowls. Join any new activity that interests you and, hopefully, you will awake the passions of someone who shares the same interests as you.

Don't assume that because you are in your fifties you can only attract someone in their fifties or older. The odds are they are only interested in a twenty-five-year-old. This is the age of the older woman with a younger man. So don't dismiss someone who is much younger than you. I like Marianne Faithfull's yardstick. When asked if she was likely to pull one of the guys in the band supporting her she said she drew the line at anyone younger than her son! I think that's a fantastic barometer. My yardstick is, is he a baby boomer? That's a pretty broad range!

## Pets

If you find life a little lonely because you don't have a love interest or partner, consider getting a dog. A dog won't answer back, will give you unconditional love, and will make sure you get lots of fresh air and exercise. Studies have shown that social isolation can lead to high blood pressure and obesity. Owning an animal is exceptionally good at bringing down blood pressure, increasing your levels of endorphins, and getting you out power walking your 10,000 steps. Some hospitals allow pro-active therapy (PAT) dogs in to visit their long-term elderly patients because they know how much good stroking a dog does them. Cats, horses, tortoises are all great, but a dog is an all-round anti-ager.

## Appearance

A lot of women, including me, get to middle age and suddenly find they have become invisible because of their lack of youth. I'm not suggesting for one moment that we get the hot pants out and do the very disastrous mutton dressed as lamb thing. But there is a lot we can do to make the very best first impression we can, so we are noticed for our style, femininity and amazing confidence. We have plenty of role models who look stunning and sexy without resorting to facelifts or tarty clothes – Helen Mirren and Joanna Lumley for example.

I *am* invisible when I scrape my hair back, wear no make-up, and go up the street hiding behind baggy sweats, trainers and comfy tops. If I dress like that, which I often do when I'm working hard, I look in the mirror and feel old and unattractive. And guess what? I start acting old and unattractive.

I am *not* invisible when I get my hair and nails done, put make-up on and dress in clothes that make me feel good. I look in the mirror and see someone who has made an effort and looks attractive. I smile. I walk out of the door and start smiling at other people. And they smile back and sometimes flirt! Whatever you put out, you will get right back. So think positive, dress positive and act positive and you will *feel* really positive about yourself and your image.

## TOP TIPS

*Do your own Trinny and Susannah: try on everything in the wardrobe and, with a ruthlessly honest best friend, decide what really makes you look good and what doesn't. Use the two-year rule. If you haven't worn it in the last two years, you never will. Try on the clothes you're not sure about and if they don't fit or you don't like them get rid of them. Sell them through a second-hand shop for a bit of extra money to buy something you really love. And don't say, 'I will fit into this one day', if you haven't in the last two years you probably never will! Most of us wear only 20 per cent of our wardrobe so keep the clothes that make you look and feel wonderful and get rid of the rest.*

*If you feel you need a complete makeover, you could always go to one of the shops or department stores that provide an image consultant who will help you decide which colours and styles work for you and which don't. It's worth the fee.*

*Make an appointment with a really top hairdresser. Get the best cut and colour you have ever had in your life, just this once.*

*Get a regular manicure. There are cheap nail bars all over the country now. You don't have to go for the full manicure, just a shape and polish, which should only set you back £10 or less.*

*Have a makeover. Skin tones change as we get older, so you need to change your make-up every few years to update your look. If you wear spectacles, invest in a really funky pair. It could take years off you.*

## Super Space

One of the best ways to have health, wealth and happiness in your life is to create *space*. If you are holding on to something negative, there is no room for the positive to come into your life. If you are feeling distracted and overwhelmed with work, look at your desk or office. Is stuff piled around everywhere? If your environment is cluttered and disorganized you will feel cluttered and disorganized. A cluttered home equals a cluttered mind and sometimes even a cluttered colon! When your home is a mess and you can't find things like the mobile, keys, letters, it isn't always a sign of dementia. You just need to get organized, have a special place for all the things you keep misplacing and clear the clutter.

## Feng Shui

Moving things around in your home can make it and you feel like new because it creates new energy in your life. Feng shui is the ancient Chinese practice of creating an energy flow in the home or the office, and the first step is decluttering. In order to encourage positive chi (energy) you need to get rid of obstructions. Clutter creates blockages that restrict the chi flow, making you feel reluctant to progress in every other area of your life.

Improving the flow of energy and creating good feng shui can bring about increased prosperity, better health and increased personal success. Giving things away is liberating. Hanging on to old possessions keeps us linked to our past and doesn't allow us to move on or forward. Here are a few examples of clutter:

Junk mail
Abandoned projects
Newspapers waiting for recycling

Things that need mending
Things waiting to go to the charity shop
Mail that hasn't been opened
Old presents that you hate
Things you never, ever use

All of these attract stale chi flow and, although I was deeply cynical, I have a very spooky example of how well it works for you. Mary Lambert, Feng Shui practitioner and author of *Declutter Workbook, 101 Steps to Transform Your Life*, came to visit my very uncluttered flat some time ago. She glanced at my bookshelves full of my beloved books and asked me if there were any I never took down to read. I had to admit that I kept my rows of old Penguin paperbacks because I liked the look of them, not because I would ever read them again. They were yellowing, smelly and at least twenty years old, but I couldn't part with them. She asked me to consider getting rid of this stale energy and, although it took me several weeks, I finally took two carrier bags' worth to the local charity shop. The very next day, I got my first publishing deal with Penguin! Now you may call it an extraordinary coincidence, but I have followed the principles of feng shui ever since.

When you surround yourself with things you love and *use*, they emit a vibrant energy that encourages the flow of chi to make your life joyful, happy and successful. If you surround yourself with unwanted, useless or broken items, their negative vibes will pull you down. So get rid of things that have no meaning to you. If you have a problem because they have lovely memories, but you no longer use them, take a photo of them and then give them away. You are letting go of your past life and new energy will come flooding into your new life, as it did mine. Here's an easy check list to find out whether it's time to let go of that clutter and encourage a little abundance into your life.

## IS IT JUNK?

- *It's broken and can't be fixed*
- *I don't like it*

- *It was an unwanted present*
- *It's out of date*
- *It doesn't fit*
- *I'm waiting to be slim enough to get into it!*

## KEEP IT IF

- *I look at it with love and feel good about it*
- *It's something I really enjoy using or wearing*
- *It is essential for my work*

Mary has a five-bag rule for clearing out the clutter. Find five heavy duty bin liners or cardboard boxes and label them as follows:

**Junk for the dump**: there will be a recycling centre near you

**Charity or friends**: it feels so good to recycle useful items

**Repairs or alterations**: get them mended

**Sort out**: old boxes of photos and cuttings are my big things

**Transitional**: keep this bag for 6 months and if you have not missed anything in it, bin it

I can't tell you how good it feels to go round your home bagging up all those old books, photos, programmes, crockery and out-of-date food. It's liberating, cleansing and you're creating space for your approaching abundance.

There are lots of other things you can do to create a super space in your home, such as 'smudging', clapping to disperse negative energy, or just spring cleaning and moving the furniture around.

## Toxins in the Home

Sitting in front of TVs or computer monitors, we are bombarded with an electromagnetic frequency of around 100 to 160 Hz. Our brainwaves vibrate at around 8Hz. That means while we are watching TV or sitting in front of the laptop for hours, our body is exposed to frequencies that vibrate twenty times faster than our brainwaves. This results in a lack of concentration, nervousness and insomnia, as well as encouraging the body to produce free radicals.

There is a lot you can do to protect yourself from these EMFs (electromagnetic fields); there are ionizers, crystal lamps and even some crystals that bind the excessive positive ions with their negative ions and help neutralize the electro-smog in a room. I have a crystal salt lamp sitting on my desk and certainly don't suffer from the busy-brain syndrome that used to keep me awake before I got it.

There is also a list of plants recommended by NASA's Dr Bill Wolverton, as being among the best for removing indoor toxins, although *all* plants help keep the air cleaner, as I'm sure you know.

## TOP TEN TOXIN-REMOVING PLANTS

*Areca palm; humidifies the air and removes indoor toxins. Most palms are excellent air cleaners.*

*Boston fern: one of the best plants for increasing humidity and removing chemical vapours such as formaldehyde.*

*Chrysanthemum: one of the best flowering plants for removing formaldehyde, benzene and ammonia from the atmosphere.*

*Dragon tree: good for a home office as it absorbs triclorethylene and xylene from computers, printers and chipboard.*

*Gerbera: removes chemical vapours while humidifying the air.*

*Ivy: in laboratory tests, ivies rated excellent for cleaning up the air.*

*Money plant: my addition, because every home should have one to create financial abundance!*

*Peace lily: my favourite plant as it's so beautiful and also excellent for removing benzene, formaldehyde and improving the moisture in dry environments.*

*Rubber plant: especially effective at clearing formaldehyde.*

*Weeping fig: a good all-round filter.*

## Super Goals

Your dreams or your goals must be as big as you are – it doesn't help you to think small. Just as muscles that aren't exercised atrophy, our dreams, visions and desires do the same if we don't exercise them. Your vision of *your* future must be bold, daring and imaginative, if you want it to come true. You need a dream of your future so powerful that you throw the duvet off in the morning and race into the day full of excitement, just like children do.

### Setting Goals

Setting goals is one of the keys to leading the life of your dreams so now is a good time to reassess your current goals (or set original goals if you haven't already). The most common mistake is to put the goal into a future tense. The goal needs to be personalized in the *present* tense and imagined with as much precise detail as possible in order to be effective.

People make a list for the supermarket all the time, yet very few of us make a list of the really important things we want in life. A really effective way of imagining how you want your life to be is to do a dream board. Get a board from a local art shop and cut out pictures of everything you would like to have in your life: your favourite car, the type of house you'd like to live in, a job, a spiritual path, a perfect pet, a gorgeous partner. Remember, it's a *dream* board, so no holds barred. Be as superficial or as serious as you like and go into as much detail as you want. Then put it where you can look at it every day to create this new life for yourself.

Each time we repeat a particular behaviour or thought, we strengthen the associated neural pathway in our brain. You need to mentally *rehearse* living the life you want. If you visualize your dreams every day, you will build stronger neural pathways to achieving them. Think of a life you want, imagine what it would be like to have it, think about how it might come about, and then focus your mind on it regularly. Here are a couple of pointers:

**Step 1**: what would you do if the world were going to end one week from today? This is the real clue to what really matters to you.

**Step 2**: brainstorm – make a list of everything you want now, have ever wanted or may want in the future.

**Step 3**: what makes your heart sing?

## Mind Mapping

I use mind mapping when I write, and introduced readers to it in my first book, to help them decide where they wanted to spend their detox weekend. It is a very useful technique for any area of your life that needs thinking about. All you need is a sheet of paper and a pen. Sit quietly without the TV or radio on, or any other distractions, and empty your mind for five minutes. Draw a circle in the middle of the paper with six or seven branches coming out of it. Put the words PERFECT LIFE in the middle of the circle and, without giving yourself a chance to dwell on it, tap your subconscious by writing a word that immediately pops into your brain on each of the branches. You can then carry on down each branch, adding to the words. For example: I may put 'writing in a tropical paradise' as one of my main branches and then add how I can get there: house swap, rental, running a workshop, meeting someone who has one. It is like a word-association game, but reveals what your inner self really needs out of life.

So I hope I have encouraged you to get yourself on track for a truly super life. We've looked at stress busting and your spiritual health, explored health, wealth and happiness, decluttered our relationships, our homes, and even our colons, and set some real goals in every area of our lives, to keep us young, vibrant, healthy and happy. I hope this has helped you as much as it's helped me writing it.

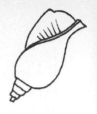

# 12.

# Super Anti-Ageing Day

This final chapter is a summary of the most important tips, techniques and exercises, as well as some new ones, to consider doing as much as possible every day as part of your anti-ageing regime. It will serve as a reminder of what to do, when you can, in the real world. There is no way you will be able to do *all* of it every day. This is, however, very much what I choose to do each day when I have the time. You may prefer to make up your own super anti-ageing day from the advice particularly pertinent to you. Or think of it as a quick checklist, in diary form, of the very best anti-ageing secrets I've shared with you and something to try out when you have a quiet weekend to concentrate on yourself.

Either way, I hope you get a lot out of this book and let me know how much younger, fitter and happier you look and feel once you've tried it all out. Here's to growing old disgracefully!

## From Getting Up to Breakfast

You should get up between 5 and 8 a.m. It is important to get up immediately you wake up, whatever the time, as long as the sun has risen. Try it for two weeks, it will take your body that long to adjust, but you will find you have a lot more energy, and time. If it's 5.30 a.m. and you think it's far too early, as long as the sun is up, it's time you were up as well. The body has had enough rest; the brain simply hasn't caught up. You need to retrain it. Have a little post-lunch nap if you are exhausted for the first couple of weeks. Eventually you will have bags more energy and time.

## Drink a Glass of Hot Water and Lemon

Squeeze half a fresh lemon into a mug of hot water and drink it. This wakes up the digestion, makes your system alkaline and is rich in vitamin C. Essential for a youthful digestion, strong immunity and clear skin.

## Move Your Bowels, If You Haven't Already!

If you want to help things along, because the soaked flaxseeds haven't kicked in yet, raise both your arms above your head. This opens up the colon and makes up for the fact that our bodies are in completely the wrong position to go to the loo. In cultures where people squat to go to the loo, colons tend to be far less sluggish. Raising your arms is almost as good as squatting.

### What Does It Look Like?

Hopefully, a perfectly smooth, brown sausage that 'hovers'. Here are a few other things to look out for.

> Pale poo means poor liver performance. Try a liver flush.
> Yellow means lymph is very active. You're detoxing.
> Floating means too much fat in the diet. Cut down on fat.
> Sinking means too much protein. Increase your fibre.
> Strong and smelly means the food hasn't been digested properly. Chew more, or take a digestive enzyme.

## Brush Teeth and Scrape Tongue

By having a quick look at your tongue every morning, before you clean your teeth, you will be able to see how your digestion is doing. If you also get into a habit of *scraping* your tongue daily you will be sending a message to your gastric juices and digestion to wake up. As soon as the millions of taste buds on your tongue are stimulated they send a message to the digestive system to get ready and your food will be broken down more efficiently.

Have a good look at your tongue. How coated is it? How white? Does your breath smell? If there is a thick white coating on the tongue, it means there is a lot of toxicity in the system, from a heavy meal or food eaten too late the night before. It could be that you are still digesting yesterday evening's food, in which case a very light breakfast or a juice would be the best thing to have to give your digestion a rest.

Use a tongue scraper (sold in health shops or by mail order) or a small spoon. Gently scrape from the back of the tongue forwards until you have scraped the whole surface. The whole process only takes twenty seconds and will get rid of that unpleasant coating, clear bacteria out of your mouth and make your breath smell sweeter!

 TOP TIP

> *Don't forget to drink 1.5–2 litres of water a day. That's one glass an hour!*

### Practise the Five Rites Exercises

These exercises only take ten minutes, once you've learned them, and are essential for anti-ageing and keeping the endocrine system healthy as well as toning the main muscle groups. They need to be done every day for maximum benefits. The exercises are described on pages 195–201.

### Skin Brush

Skin brushing is very beneficial for the lymphatic system. Using a body brush made from natural bristle, always brush in the direction the blood flows towards the heart. Brush on dry skin, starting from the soles of the feet upwards, using clockwise, circular movements. Brush the front of the body first, up to the breasts. Then start on the backs of the legs and work upwards again, until you reach the upper back. Brush downwards from the neck, towards the heart, both front and back. Finally, brush each arm from the hand up, front then back. Don't forget to brush inside your armpit, by holding the arm up and working downwards.

Don't do your face. Give the back of your neck and your scalp a good going over! You should feel very energized by the time you've done the whole body.

While you skin brush or while you prepare for your shower, empty the contents of a digestive enzyme capsule into your hands, mix with a little water and pat all over your face. Leave it on for five to ten minutes while you get on with your pre-shower bits and pieces, then wash it off.

If you don't have any digestive enzymes, freshly squeezed lemon juice is just as good as a skin brightener and natural fruit acid, but only leave it on for a couple of minutes before washing it off.

## Shower

In the shower apply a hot flannel over your face to open up the pores, then splash it with cold water or toner after your shower using rosewater. If you are washing your hair, use two whipped up egg yolks for a natural shine and conditioner.

When you have reached the end of your shower turn it on as cold as you can stand it for ten seconds (building up to thirty seconds), then turn it up to warm again for a minute or two. Repeat this three or four times and end on cool. This will boost your immune system and get your lymph moving.

## After Your Shower

Moisturize your body and face, using a rejuvenation oil and your chosen essential oils from page 177, or my recipe for an oil on page 180. If you are using wild yam cream, apply the prescribed amount to a fleshy part of the body. Stroke some pure vitamin C round the mouth or any lined area of the face.

## From Breakfast to Lunchtime

This is what I eat every morning and, amazingly, I never get bored with it. But go ahead and choose whatever you like from Super Foods on page 150.

Mix the following ingredients into 125g of live goat's yogurt.

2 tablespoons soaked wolfberries, or any other berries
1 dessertspoon soaked flaxseeds
2 teaspoons bee pollen
2 heaped teaspoons maca
1 teaspoon lecithin granules

### Start 10,000 Steps

Whether you are walking part of the way to work, walking your dog, or simply getting out for some fresh air this is your chance to get at least 5,000 steps under your belt. Take small steps and you will accomplish half your daily requirement more easily. At the same time you will be getting some vitamin D, for calcium absorption, encouraging your body to produce more of the anti-ageing hormone, GH, and helping to prevent osteoporosis.

I walk along the promenade every day, come hail or shine, and cannot start work without doing this first. Take a Walkman or an iPod to listen or dance along to; or take some time out for a 'quiet' time.

This is also the perfect chance to get some light into the pineal gland and do a quick breathing exercise/meditation at the same time. Leave your mobile turned off and take your sunglasses off, so the light goes through your retina into the pineal gland.

## Lunch

This should be the biggest meal of the day and eaten as early as noon and no later than 2 p.m.

On page 227 is what I typically eat for lunch, when I am working at home. It won't suit anyone working away from home unless you take it in with you.

Before lunch, drink a glass of vegetable juice or eat a handful of 'living' alfalfa sprouts, or similar.

## BIG SALAD WITH SUZI'S DRESSING

*big handful of alfalfa sprouts*
*200g mixed salad leaves: rocket, spinach and watercress*
*1 small avocado*
*raw carrot or beetroot, grated*
*1 dessertspoon mixed seeds*

for the dressing
*1 teaspoon olive oil*
*2–3 teaspoons omega-3 and 6 oil, such as flaxseed or hempseed*
*1 dessertspoon lemon juice*
*1 small clove garlic, crushed*
*1 teaspoon mayonnaise*
*pinch of salt (unrefined sea or crystal)*

Put the salad ingredients into a bowl. Mix all the dressing ingredients together, pour over the salad and toss well. You can add seeds, pine nuts or one of the permitted cheeses making it a complete, protein-rich meal. Add some oily fish for added omega-3 benefits and you still have a meal that is 80 per cent raw and living. If it's winter I might have quinoa with this salad to make it a little more filling.

With lunch take 6 spirulina tablets for extra energy and anti-ageing nutrients, 2 homocysteine-lowering supplements and 2 1000mg fish-oil capsules.

## From Lunch to Supper

Have a post-lunch rest at about 2 o'clock. This is the usual time for our natural body rhythms to slow right down as the pineal gland releases smaller amounts of melatonin. Have a catnap of no more than fifteen minutes, if you can, to allow your digestion to do its job properly. This will not throw your body clock out of synch or prevent you from sleeping at night.

However, if you are working you can't do this, unless you sneak off to the loo! Make sure to sit quietly for at least five minutes after eating rather than bolting your food down at your desk and immediately rushing about.

## Walking

Walk more of your steps, if you can. Walking for five to fifteen minutes after lunch aids digestion.

## Afternoon Snack

An apple
A few soaked, mixed nuts: walnuts, hazelnuts and pecans
A mug of green tea

You should have moved your bowels again, by now!

## Walking

Try and complete your 10,000 steps, by walking back from work, or to the shops, or going to the park.

## Meditation

 TOP TIPS

*Start with five minutes a day*
*Have a focal point such as a flower, tree, candle or statue*
*Use ear plugs if it's noisy*
*Wear loose, comfortable clothes*
*Face east if you can*
*Keep your eyes closed*
*Look at an imaginary white light between the eyes*
*Play New-Age music if it helps*

Take your shoes off. Sit cross-legged on the floor. If you have trouble keeping your spine straight, sit with your back against a wall or in a chair, as long as it is straight-backed and your feet are resting comfortably on the floor. Have your palms facing up and open like empty bowls, on your knees. Close your eyes. Keep them relaxed and imagine there is a white dot between your eyebrows.

Breathe normally, but gradually begin to notice your breathing. Don't try and influence it in any way, just observe it. Allow it to reach its own rhythm.

If your brain starts getting busy and you start making lists, don't try and stop it. Look at the thought, imagine it in a bubble and blow it away. Then come back to watching your breathing. It is a very simple exercise but takes practice to get used to 'watching' those thoughts, letting go of them and getting back into stillness and nothingness. But with practice, it will come.

At the end of your meditation, sit quietly and let your body come back to the present. You will feel so relaxed and energized you will wonder why you have never done it before! It is a wonderful technique to use if you come home exhausted, wondering how you are going to keep going through the evening. Try it for just five minutes.

## From Supper to Bedtime

### Supper

This is always my smallest meal of the day, unless I'm going out for dinner. I usually have a pint glass of vegetable juice made up of:

> 4 carrots
> 1 small beetroot
> 2 sticks celery
> ¼ cucumber
> 1 apple or small orange to sweeten
> a chunk of ginger

or a shot of wheatgrass and orange, followed by two big spelt, seeded crackers with hummus, spicy pinto or tahini paste, covered with avocado and alfalfa sprouts and sprinkled with nori flakes.

This is usually enough for me, but I do have days when I need more food, especially in the winter or if I haven't had a big lunch. More fish or a curry will usually hit the spot!

If I am going out for dinner, I swap the meals around and have a light lunch and what I like in the evening.

## After Supper

Rest for five minutes, then have a walk to aid digestion for fifteen minutes.

## Evening Bath

If you are spending a quiet evening in, this is the perfect opportunity to try an Epsom salt bath and follow it with a full body massage.

The temperature should be as hot as is comfortable. Add 1 cup of Epsom salts to a full bath and soak for ten to twenty minutes. Epsom salts are quite detoxing so only have these baths on three consecutive nights, then normal baths.

While you are in the bath you can exfoliate and use a facemask. I usually do this once a week.

### Exfoliator

Mix a little with extra virgin olive oil or one of the other oils (see page 176) with an unrefined, unprocessed sea or crystal salt. Rub the mixture gently all over your body and face, using circular motions.

### Anti-Ageing Facemask

Mash a ripe avocado and add fresh squeezed lemon juice and a little of your chosen carrier oil. Smother your face with this delicious-tasting concoction and cover your eyes with cucumber circles, taken straight from the fridge.

*Full Body Massage*

After your bath, wrap up warmly and rest for a few minutes. Put 1–2 tablespoons of carrier oil into a little bowl, add 3–6 drops of your chosen essential oil and mix. You could also fill a little plastic bottle with a carrier oil and then add 5–10 drops of essential oil, giving the bottle a good shake every time you self-massage.

Here's a reminder of the best anti-ageing and essential oils.

## CARRIER OILS

- *Flaxseed*
- *Argan*
- *Grapeseed*
- *Olive*

## ESSENTIAL OILS

- *Rose Absolute: for mature skin*
- *Benzoin: tightens skin*
- *Myrrh: firms saggy skin*
- *Frankincense: skin-cell regenerator*
- *Lavender: the relaxer (not that you will need it after that bath!)*
- *Lemon: stimulates new cells*

Some of you may be familiar with this massage from my first book; it was given to me by masseuse Janie Hildebrand.

It is important to always work towards the heart because you are helping the lymph move. Work from the head down and from the legs and stomach up just as you do with body brushing, but this time starting with the head.

Slowly 'shampoo' your scalp all over using the pads of your fingers, not your nails, working the oil well into the scalp. This movement is incredibly relaxing as well as being very good for your hair. Leave the oil on your scalp.

Using the pads of the fingers and thumbs, gently pinch the skin of the face. Moving in small, circular movements work up over the cheeks, working deeply as if kneading dough! Work up over the forehead until the whole face has been kneaded. This is really good for getting deep into the facial tissue increasing circulation, lymphatic drainage and elasticity.

Move down to the neck and shoulders. With a well-oiled hand, pinch the flesh on top of your shoulder blade between the first three fingers and thumb of your opposite hand, moving up and down the entire length of each shoulder. And then, with one hand, very gently massage the back of your neck. Or get someone to do it for you!

Try and cup your whole arm by placing your fingers on top and your thumb underneath. Start at the wrist and, using upward strokes, glide up your arm pressing firmly. Repeat several times on each arm alternating between thumb on top and thumb underneath.

Move on to your feet. Sit down and put a foot on the opposite knee. Nestle your toes in your hand, and with your other hand, using only your knuckles, circle all over the bottom of your foot. Squeeze the back and sides above the heel, where a lot of tension is held. Finish by pulling each toe gently but briskly, making sure each one is oiled. Repeat on the other foot.

With one foot on the side of the bath, cup both your hands round your leg. Work from above the anklebone, firmly and slowly gliding both hands up the leg and over the knee. You might have to do this several times to make sure your whole leg has been massaged. Re-oil your hands and do the same to your thigh, but this time using more pressure. Repeat on the other side.

Finally, floss and *then* brush the teeth with an electric toothbrush.

By now you should be ready for bed and a fantastic regenerating night's sleep. Sleep well.

# Resources

## Further Reading

Braverman, Eric R., *The Edge Effect* (Sterling Publishing)

Budwig, Dr Johanna, *Flax Oil as a True Aid Against Arthritis, Heart Infarction, Cancer and Other Diseases* (Apple Publishing)

Buzan, Tony, *The Mind Map Book* (BBC)

Christy, Martha M., *Your Own Perfect Medicine* (Wishland Publishing)

Clement, Brian R., *Living Foods for Optimum Health* (Prima Publishing)

Durrant-Peatfield, Dr Barry, *The Great Thyroid Scandal and How to Survive It* (Barons Down Publishing)

Erasmus, Udo, *Fats That Heal, Fats That Kill* (Alive Books)

——, *Choosing the Right Fats* (Alive Books)

Holford, Patrick, and Braly, James, *The H Factor Solution* (Basic Health Publications)

Lambert, Mary, *Declutter Workbook: 101 Steps to Transform Your Life* (Cico Books)

Millstone, Erik, and Lang, Tim, *The Atlas of Food: Who Eats What, Where and Why* (Earthscan Publications)

Patterson, Conor, *Aim for the Stars, Reach for the Moon* (O Books)

## Organizations and Experts

Suzi Grant: *www.suzigrant.com*

British Association for Nutritional Therapy: *www.bant.org.uk*

Allergy UK: *www.allergyuk.org* tel: 01322 619864

Professor Loren Cordain, PhD, Department of Health and Exercise Science, Colorado State University: *www.thepaleodiet.com*

Hippocrates Health Institute: *www.hippocratesinst.org*
Dr Nicholas Perricone: *www.nvperriconemd.co.uk*
Homocysteine testing, York Test Laboratories: *www.yorktest.com*
  tel: 0800 0746185
Eye health: *www.eyesight.nu* tel: 0870 241 4237
Breast Health: Bristol Cancer Help Centre, *www.bristolcancerhelp.*
  *org* tel: 0845 1232311
Incontinence: *www.continence-foundation.org.uk* tel: 0845 345 0165
BMI index: *www.bbc.co.uk/health/yourweight/bmi.shtml*
Isolagen: *www.isolagen.co.uk*
Cleo II Facial Exerciser: *www.club-cleo.com*
Tai Chi website: *www.taichifinder.co.uk*
Open University: *www.open.ac.uk* tel: 0870 33 33 43 40
Mary Lambert: *www.marylambertfengshui.com*
For facial acupuncture: *www.acupuncture.org.uk*
Julia Hancock: *www.fracupuncture.co.uk.*
Conor Patterson: *www.lifecoach.gb.com*
Janie Hildebrand: *www.janie@janiehealer.com*

## Suppliers

For tasteless flaxseed oil, lecithin and EPA fish-oil capsules:
  *www.nutrigold.co.uk* tel: 01884 251 777.
For argan oil: *www.wildwoodgroves.com*, Wild Wood Groves is
  committed to providing fair trade employment in its oil production and contributing to the conservation of the argan tree.
Water, under sink, counter and portable systems: Wellness Water,
  *www.wellness-water.co.uk*
Udo's Choice oil blend & Digestive Enzymes: Savant Distribution,
  *www.savant-health.com* tel: 08450 60 60 70
Maca, bee pollen, wolfberries & essential oils: *www.tree-harvest.com*
  tel: 01531 65 07 64
Homocysteine and heart nutrients, H Factors (put together by
  Patrick Holford): Higher Nature, *www.highernature.co.uk* tel:
  01435 884668
Immun'Age: *www.immunage.info*

Spirulina: *www.hawaiianspirulina.com*

For wild yam products: *www.natural-woman.com* tel: 0117 968 7744

Himalayan crystal salt & crystal salt lamps: *www.bestcareproducts. com*

For vitamin C ester and vitamin E in liquid form: *www.biocare. co.uk* tel: 0121 433 3727

Masai Barefoot Technology: *www.mbt-uk.com*

# Index